Transition from Student Nurse to
REGISTERED NURSE

A Guide to Help You
Navigate Through
Nursing Better

1ST EDITION

JJ Cai Junjie, RN, BSc (Nursing) (Hons), GC-WOCP
Registered Nurse, Singapore Nursing Board;
Bachelor of Science (Nursing) (Honours),
National University of Singapore;
Graduate Certification in Wound, Ostomy,
and Continence Practice,
Curtin University

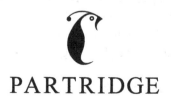

PARTRIDGE

Library of Congress Control Number: 2018943924
ISBN: Hardcover   978-1-5437-4553-5
               Softcover   978-1-5437-4551-1
               eBook   978-1-5437-4552-8

Print information available on the last page.

To order additional copies of this book, contact
Toll Free 800 101 2657 (Singapore)
Toll Free 1 800 81 7340 (Malaysia)
orders.singapore@partridgepublishing.com

www.partridgepublishing.com/singapore

CONTENTS

Section 1: Clinical Years

Section 2: Transition-to-Practice

LIST OF TABLES

LIST OF FIGURES

PREFACE

In the years while deciding to join Nursing and even after I have become a Registered Nurse, I have heard many of my family members, colleagues, friends and even strangers talk about what they think of this career. Some hold it in high regard, some are exaggerated while others are just demeaning. While Nursing can be a deeply rewarding career, I have also seen some of my friends and colleagues leave this profession because they were unable to align with the demands of this job.

I believe that Nursing can be enjoyed and not just endured. If you can see what this job offers, then you have found the pot of gold at the end of the rainbow. However, some navigation may be required.

And that is the reason behind the creation of this book!

To figure out ways to smoothen the transition from a student to a Registered Nurse, I have gathered some questions that our budding student nurses wished they knew before they headed out to the "real world". I have also gathered feedback and opinions of those that have gone into this profession to find out the things that they wished they had known before they started working.

I hope that this book will find you well. It will be my pleasure to revise this book to continue to meet your needs as a nursing student, nursing graduate, or even as a seasoned practising nurse.

JJ Cai Junjie
REGISTERED NURSE

DEDICATION

To Dr. Liaw Sok Ying, my teacher, mentor, and the one who encouraged me to turn this guide into a book and reality. I would have never imagined myself be able to write a book without her encouragement. Thank you for introducing me to Ms. Wong Lai Fun who passionately helped with editing and providing countless valuable advice to make this guide into a refined piece.

To my family, who believed in me even before I have accomplished anything, I love you all.

To Rebecca, who never once despised my initial raw ideas and through your words of wisdom, have made this book into an even better piece. I am excited to continue journeying through life with you!

To my nursing peers, juniors, non-nursing mentors, and friends, thank you for all the kind words. Your kind words have given me the confidence to continue writing.

To Leo Qian Wen, Joanne Seah Kwang Hui, and Daniel Chee Guang Hui, thank you to all of you for the support as (then) students to give critiques and affirmations, to generate ideas, and make this book a far better piece and a reality!

Lastly, to God who is the true Creator of everything, and who made everything possible and beautiful in its time!

CONTRIBUTORS & REVIEWERS

Wong Lai Fun
Lecturer
National University of Singapore, Alice Lee Centre of Nursing
Studies

Dr. Rebecca Goh Wenhui
BMBS (University of Southampton)
MMedSc (University of Southampton)

Dr. Ryan Tan Choon Kiat
MBBS (National University of Singapore)
Member of the Royal College of Surgeons (Ireland)

Dr. Tang Si Zhao
MD (National University of Malaysia)
PgCert (Edinburgh)

Matthew Neo Ji Hui
Bachelor of Applied Science (Physiotherapy) (Honours I)
University of Sydney

Chew Tee Kit
Bachelor of Arts (Social Work)
National University of Singapore

Hoong Jian Ming
Bachelor of Health Science (Nutrition and Dietetics) (Honours)
Queensland University of Technology

Katherine Lim Ci Hui
BSc (Nursing) (Honours) (National University of Singapore)
Specialist Diploma in Palliative Care Nursing (Ngee Ann Polytechnic)

Janice Tang Si Jia
Bachelor of Speech Pathology (Honours)
The University of Queensland

Timothy Koh Yi Kiet
Bachelor of Science (Pharmacy) (Honours)
National University of Singapore

Acacia Neo Jia Wei
Bachelor of Health Science (Podiatry) (Honours)
Queensland University of Technology

Chan Jingyi Priscilla
Bachelor of Science (Occupational Therapy)
Trinity College Dublin

Tan Kai Beng
Bachelor of Science (Nursing) (Honours)
National University of Singapore

INTRODUCTION

This book is divided into two sections—Clinical Years and Transition-to-Practice.

Clinical Years introduces the complex yet enriching world of nursing by presenting an overview of our present-day local healthcare system. This section offers you the compass to navigate through the system with the right learning approach towards nursing. This is achieved through the laying down of the fundamentals clearly and firmly for you, the student nurse/ novice nurse, to build upon as you approach your transition to the working world.

Transition-to-Practice further equips you with practical and applicable knowledge and tips to tread through the murky waters with greater confidence. It is my hope that, at the end of the journey, you will be ready to receive the mantle of a registered nurse (RN).

This book focuses mainly on transiting the student nurse into the general ward more so than in other areas of nursing care. This is because most students start off their journey by having their transition-to-practice in the general ward rather than in specialised areas such as in the operating theatres, intensive care unit, or the community. It will be, however, my greatest delight to eventually write more content for transition into other areas in the future. In the meantime, please enjoy this carefully arranged book!

SECTION I

CLINICAL YEARS

We begin our nursing journey when we start to meet real patients in the different settings where we are not *directly responsible* for their care, but as *bystanders*. We gain clarity when we try to figure out what is going on, to have some practice while not getting in the way, and answering this very important question in our heads: *What would I do if I am the staff nurse in-charge of this patient?*

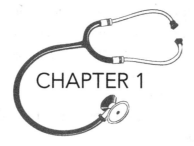

CHAPTER 1

TYPES OF HEALTHCARE DELIVERY

One of the extremely important things we need to know before we head out for our clinical placements is to know *where* we are going to carry out the duties. Every healthcare setting presents different nursing needs and learning opportunities. Therefore, it is important to understand how the healthcare system works in Singapore by breaking it down. There are three main categories[1]:

- Primary healthcare services (e.g. Polyclinics, General Practices)
- Secondary/tertiary services (e.g. Restructured Hospitals)
- Intermediate and long-term care (ILTC) services (e.g. Nursing Homes, Home Nursing Services)

As you can see, the classical classification model (primary to tertiary healthcare) has been modified in our country in order to meet the demands of the ageing population. As a nursing student/nursing graduate in Singapore, you should be exposed to the different healthcare delivery systems to have a clearer picture of how the systems serve its population.

---

[1] Ministry of Health Singapore, "Healthcare Services and Facilities," last modified July 31, 2018, https://www.moh.gov.sg/our-healthcare-system/healthcare-services-and-facilities.

Most schools, at least for Alice Lee Centre for Nursing Studies (ALCNS), prefer sending their students to ILTC services and primary healthcare services before secondary and tertiary institutions. Restructured hospitals tend to be a more challenging and fast-paced environment due to the acuity of the patients' conditions.

Here is a general breakdown of the healthcare delivery system in Singapore.

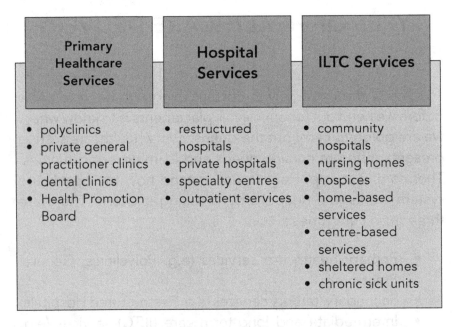

Primary Healthcare Services	Hospital Services	ILTC Services
• polyclinics • private general practitioner clinics • dental clinics • Health Promotion Board	• restructured hospitals • private hospitals • specialty centres • outpatient services	• community hospitals • nursing homes • hospices • home-based services • centre-based services • sheltered homes • chronic sick units

Table 1.1 Three Main Categories of
Healthcare Delivery in Singapore

Most of the intensive learning comes from restructured hospitals. In fact, the Singapore Nursing Board (SNB) has a set of requirements that each nursing student needs to complete prior to becoming a registered nurse (RN). These learning opportunities to fulfil these requirements are usually only found in restructured hospitals due to the large volume of patients with more acute conditions.

In the next few pages, some of the insights and expectations on the different healthcare delivery settings will be revealed to you.

PRIMARY HEALTHCARE SERVICES

Here, you will be posted to the polyclinics to observe or participate in some of the services that are available:

- Doctor's consultation for minor ailments and beyond (e.g. upper respiratory tract infection)
- Screening for diseases like diabetes, colon cancers, and cervical cancers
- Chronic disease management (counselling, education, follow-up, and screening for complications like diabetic foot neuropathy)
- Vaccinations (adults and children)
- Monitoring children's developmental growth
- Lifestyle and diet modification and counselling (e.g. smoking cessation)
- Simple wound dressings, STO (suture to off)
- Minor surgical procedures (e.g. wedge resection of ingrown toenail)

A great emphasis is placed on disease prevention, treatment of milder diseases, and the follow-up care and monitoring after the acute phase of disease. These allow members of the public to be cared for at the *community level*.

HOSPITAL SERVICES

Here, you will be attached to the various restructured hospitals and possibly specialty centres (skin, heart, cancer, neuroscience, and dental centres). Patients who require admission to hospital services for treatment of acute conditions and round-the-clock medical, nursing, and allied health attention will be taken care of at these places. Below are some services provided at the hospital:

- **Emergency Medicine.** This department mainly deals with cases involving cardiac/pulmonary/neurological/ haemodynamic compromises/instabilities at the initial phase. For instance, cases seen would be road traffic accidents, acute myocardial infarctions, and intra-cranial haemorrhages. It also includes triaging to determine the severity of cases in order to prioritise their care. Critically-ill patients may be haemodynamically stable on arrival but present with symptoms such as persistent pain. The department determines whether a patient needs admission to the hospital.

- **Intensive Care Medicine.** Critically-ill patients who require intensive management and close monitoring are admitted to this discipline. These patients may require mechanical ventilation, intra-arterial line, and constant nursing monitoring. The gist of the discipline is close monitoring until patients are out of the critical phase. Examples of these cases are the post-cardiac arrest patient, post-major surgery patient, and massive trauma patient.

- **General Surgery.** General surgical cases that require surgical intervention are admitted to this discipline. Common invasive procedures and surgeries seen are colonoscopy, incision and drainage of abscesses, laparoscopic or open (laparotomy) exploration of the abdominal cavity, and appendectomy. More specific subspecialties of General Surgery include Vascular Surgery (e.g., angiogram/angioplasty and creation of arteriovenous fistula), Colorectal Surgery (e.g., intestinal resections that may involve stoma creation), and Upper Gastrointestinal Surgery (e.g. reflux, bariatric surgery). There is a move towards admitting patients under an acute care surgery team (ACS) which sees generic surgical conditions, before eventually allocating patients requiring subspecialty attention to the relevant subspecialties such as Colorectal, Hepatobiliary, or Upper Gastrointestinal Surgery.

- **Orthopaedics.** This department sees conditions involving disorders of the musculoskeletal system, like abscess of the limbs and tibia fractures. In our aging population, hip fractures are one of the most common causes for admission to the Orthopaedics department. More specific subspecialisation includes foot and ankle, spine, hand and reconstructive microsurgery. A patient with a slipped disc requiring discectomy, for instance, would be taken care of by the Spine Surgery team—a subspecialty of Orthopaedics.

- **Medicine.** In Singapore, the bulk of hospital admissions are under General Medicine, also known as Internal Medicine. Many restructured hospitals have a practice of admitting patients that are assessed to have non-complex needs and an estimated short inpatient stay under the Acute Internal Medicine (AIM) teams. Some of such common presentations include chronic obstructive pulmonary disease (COPD) exacerbation, asthma exacerbation, uncomplicated hypo/hyperglycaemia, and cellulitis. Other subspecialisations can include Respiratory Medicine (e.g. cystic fibrosis and pulmonary tuberculosis), Endocrinology (e.g., hypo/hyperthyroidism and uncontrolled diabetes), Renal Medicine (e.g., acute kidney failures and dialysis-related issues or dialysis support), and Infectious Diseases (infections involving multidrug resistant microbes, highly infectious diseases, and advice on more complicated antibiotic treatment).

- **Cardiology and Cardiothoracic Vascular Surgery (CTVS).** Cardiac conditions that do not require surgery, like heart failures and ischaemic heart disease, are managed under Cardiology. On the other hand, patients who require percutaneous coronary interventions, coronary bypasses, and heart transplants will be taken care of under the CTVS discipline, along with other heart issues that may require surgery.
- **Neurology and Neurosurgery.** Neurological issues, like seizures and breakthrough seizures, are classified under the Neurology department. However, issues like subdural haemorrhage (requiring craniotomy) and brain aneurysm (requiring endovascular coiling) would be classified under Neurosurgery, as they require surgical interventions.
- **Obstetrics and Gynaecology (O&G).** Problems pertaining to the female reproductive system, including childbearing, are taken care of in this department. Pre/postpartum problems like preeclampsia and postpartum bleeding would be classified under Obstetrics. Non-pregnancy related conditions such as cancers of the cervix or uterus, or menstrual disorders, are managed by the Gynaecology department.
- **Paediatrics.** All medical and surgical cases involving children below the age of eighteen are to be seen in the Paediatrics department. Subspecialisations mirror various aspects of the adult health as the physiology of an infant, toddler, and adolescent vary much from an adult.
- **Psychiatry.** Patients with mental disorders/issues, such as schizophrenia, major depressive disorders, and obsessive-compulsive disorders are to be seen by the Psychiatrist. Typically, mental disorders warranting admission would need to be of a greater acuity. They would be or at a potential of causing self-harm or harm

to people around them or they are highly dysfunctional and disruptive in the community. Such cases may require admission to the Institute of Mental Health (IMH).

This list, however, is *not exhaustive*. It is listed extensively to provide a rough idea of the common issues you might encounter as you step into the hospital. This will assist in your preparation for these clinical postings and/or working life.

To help your learning further, I will also explain this interesting referral system called the *blue letter*. These referrals are known as blue letters because such referrals were traditionally written on blue-coloured letters for the medical and healthcare teams to differentiate them from the progress notes. Interestingly, even after the introduction of electronic documentation, the term "blue letter" has still been retained in our local hospitals.

In day-to-day operations, a medical team caring for a particular patient may realise that they require input from other disciplines as newer or multiple issues arise since our organ systems are linked. Blue letters are internal referrals within the hospital from one speciality to another. For instance, an Orthopaedic Surgery patient with an infected wound of the lower limb that is healing poorly may be referred to the Vascular Surgery team to evaluate for peripheral arterial disease which may be impairing the wound's healing. The Orthopaedics Surgery team may also refer to Cardiology to assess for cardiac risks for subsequent surgery because of the patient's multiple cardiac co-morbidities, such as smoking and a previous history of ischaemic heart disease.

Types of Nursing Services

The classification of different medical and surgical problems and how care is being transferred from one provider to another will take you some time to get used to it. Along with the understanding of how care can be co-managed by different medical specialties, you will also understand that sometimes nursing care involves specialty nurses to provide a particular type of care.

Specialty Care/Advanced Practice Nurse (APN)

The role of the APN and specialty care nurse is to provide specialised or higher level of care and counselling for patients and caregivers. He/she can function independently as well as in collaboration with the multidisciplinary team. Certain conditions require patients and their caregivers to adjust, adapt, and follow through their new conditions to effectively manage their health back at home.

I will list a few common specialties in the next two pages that are usually offered in our restructured hospitals. Please bear in mind that they are *not exhaustive*.

Diabetes Nurse Educator (DNE)

The DNE is the specialist nurse who manages patients with newly diagnosed or poorly controlled diabetes. DNEs will educate these patients and their caregivers on the disease process, treatment, and preventive measures for development of complications. They often counsel patients on the following issues:

- Insulin injection technique
- Use of blood glucose device
- Monitoring of blood glucose levels
- Diet counselling
- Advice for sick days and during fasting months
- Advice for regular foot and eye screening

For patients who are newly started on insulin injections during their admission, the DNE is the one to go to for clearance of the insulin injection technique and subsequent monitoring of blood sugar levels. In some settings, the DNE will also be able to titrate insulin doses with an Endocrinologist.

Pain Management Nurse

This is a nurse specialised in managing pain, ranging from acute to chronic pain. The Pain Management Nurse is able to titrate analgesia and provide suggestions for the appropriate mode and dose of analgesia that would be suitable for the patient's condition, his background and underlying medical comorbidities. Such analgesia may come in the form of oral, intravenous, topical or injections. Pain Management Nurses often work closely with the Anaesthetists, some of whom also choose to subspecialise in Pain Management.

Palliative Care Nurse

This is a nurse specialised in looking into the needs and comfort of patients at the end of life. This includes the management of uncomfortable symptoms such as pain and shortness of breath, as part of the disease process. It is common that spiritual needs and wishes of the dying patient are not adequately met in the acute hospitals because our main goal of care is often to take care of the patient so that he/she is fit to be discharged. It is essential that there are healthcare providers that look into such needs where medical science fails to treat.

Furthermore, patients and caregivers may not be ready to accept being diagnosed as terminally ill, especially if the underlying disease process such as cancer is not discovered until their admission. Counselling and end-of-life care discussions are often needed so that the process of grief can be complete and the suffering be kept to a minimum.

Wound Care Nurse

Advancement in wound treatment modalities has created a great need for nurses with the knowledge and ability to manage complex wounds. These nurses can perform negative pressure wound therapy and select from a great range of wound products to tackle different types of wounds. They are key resource personnel for consultation should the wound be complex, requiring thorough examination and assessment for potential complications, or failing to improve despite simple topical dressings.

They often work closely with the various Surgical disciplines and in some settings may also be able to perform conservative bedside sharp wound debridement.

Stoma Care/Enterostomal Therapy Nurse

Having a stoma, be it temporary or permanent, can be very distressing due to the appearance and smell of the discharges from the stoma. If stoma siting is not done *prior to* operation, the eventual stoma position may not be ideal for the adherence of stoma appliances. This could make the management of stoma contents extremely challenging. Enterostomal therapy nurses play a key role in providing care and training to the patients and their caregivers so that living with a stoma can be less of a challenge. Stoma Care nurses work closely with the General Surgery team, especially the Colorectal team, in the care of patients with stomas.

ILTC SERVICES

Here, you will be visiting the community hospitals, hospices, and possibly home-based services.

Community Hospitals

Community hospitals, one of the services in residential ILTC, care for patients who are medically stable, but still require continual medical, nursing, and rehabilitation care for a short period of time.

Common problems that patients have in the community hospitals are post-limb amputations (with or without wound infections), post-fractures, post-stroke, difficult to treat infections, and post-operative deconditioning. These problems can potentially take weeks to months to fully recover. Admitting these patients into the community hospitals or enrolling them in day-care and ancillary programs in the community can then help decongest the usually packed acute hospitals. Community hospitals can also accept patients that require respite or interim care on a case-by-case basis.

For instance, the patients in the community hospital may require:

- **Intravenous (IV) antibiotic therapy.** For patients who require the completion of antibiotic therapy and have no suitable oral alternatives, they require the aid of RNs for IV access and administration of IV medication. While outpatient antibiotics therapy (OPAT) service is a popular choice, some patients who are not ambulatory enough may have difficulties in arranging daily trips to the hospital or they do not qualify to utilise the OPAT services due to financial reasons.
- **Wound care.** More complicated wounds may require more extensive treatment and vigilant monitoring. The use of negative pressure wound therapy (NPWT) is an example. NPWT can be continued at home, but if patients are not able to handle NPWT safely, community hospital or home nursing services must be considered.
- **Rehabilitation.** Patients who experienced medical events such as a major operation and prolonged bed-rest due to critical illness may have extensive muscle wastage. They may not be safe to be discharged back home straight from the acute hospital. Those identified to have a

potentially good recovery prognosis will undergo intensive rehabilitation at the community hospital with the aim of optimising their functional outcome before returning home. Rehabilitation programmes are individualised and delivered by the physiotherapist (PT) and/or occupational therapist (OT) in the community hospitals.

Hospices

Hospices are for patients who have a prognosis of **three months** or less. Most of these patients may have symptoms or nursing needs that may be stressful and demanding for caregivers to manage at home as the patients' diseases progress. These patients may experience the following:

- Shortness of breath (SOB)
- Delirium
- Severe pain
- Fungating wounds

They may require a 24-hour caregiver, high-volume supplemental oxygen, pain medications that require titration, continuous nutritional support and/or complex wound care. In such situations, patients could benefit from inpatient stay, as their caregivers may not have the resources or knowledge to fully care for them at home.

Centre-Based/Community-Based Services

Some patients who are community-ambulant with manageable conditions but do not need a 24-hour caregiver may consider centre-based services. These services can include day care, dementia day care, and hospice day care. In addition, there are also day rehabilitation services which offer maintenance physiotherapy and occupational therapy for patients after they have been discharged from a Restructured Hospital or Community Hospital. There is also a new programme called Integrated Home and Day-Care Services (IHDC) which provides both home care and day care services for patients with higher care needs.

Home-Based Services

In view of hospital bed-crunches and rising healthcare costs, there has been a greater push for more home-based services to help patients stay in their communities by managing their activities of daily living (ADLs), basic care, and chronic conditions better. This reduces the frequency of hospital visits and avoids inpatient stay. Some of these services, ranging from simple non-medical/nursing tasks to complex medical/ nursing assessments, may include:

- Assistance with ADLs (e.g., showering)
- Medical escort services
- Meals delivery
- Chronic wound care
- Stoma care
- Routine change of naso-gastric tube
- Routine change of urinary indwelling catheter
- Home nurse visits to monitor and improve medication compliance
- Palliative/end-of-life care with home visits
- Doctor's review of chronic diseases
- Physiotherapy and occupational therapy rehabilitation

Note: Home hospice services would require patients to have a prognosis of *less than one year*.

These services are now evolving so that stable patients with higher care needs can be managed in the community or at home instead. Even complex treatments like chemotherapy are now being piloted at the community level. More complex home-based services can be expected in the near future as more advanced community care programmes are being developed.

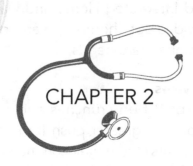

CHAPTER 2

LEARNING IN ACUTE SETTINGS

The acute settings provide the most plentiful opportunities for acquiring nursing skills and knowledge. However, you may find that resources for learning may not be equally distributed among different settings, or even among nursing students. Your friend's preceptor or clinical instructor may seem to be more nurturing than yours, or you may feel that your preceptor has something against you and you may find him/her not as approachable as you hoped. These are simply just real-world problems.

Nevertheless, here are some tips to help you maximise your learning even in the most unstructured setting that you are attached to.

Be Prepared

- Research on the discipline that you will be posted to. Have a knowledge of the common medical and nursing problems related to the discipline and a brief understanding of how these issues are managed.
- Arrive early to read about the existing treatment and nursing care plans for the patients you are assigned to for your shift.

- Plan and write out the questions to ask at the end of the shift. Clarify questions that require more explanation at the next possible timing with your preceptor.

Be Curious

- Correlate the patient's condition with the existing medical treatment and nursing care plans.
- Draw similarities and differences between the treatment plans of patients. Attempt to rationalise.
- Question and even challenge the existing plans.

Be Proactive

- Help with daily routines/activities of daily living (ADL) in the ward—hygiene, elimination, ambulation, and diet serving. By helping, you get to practise basic nursing skills and it will also free up your preceptor's time. This will make it easier for your preceptor to set aside time to have discussions with you, supervise your procedures and to simply teach you.
- Participate in the clinical activities that your assigned staff nurse or preceptor is doing. However, your assigned staff nurse usually expects the daily needs to be taken care of (especially the morning routines) before you can join him/her in medication serving or in performing nursing procedures.

Be Positive

- It is okay if things do not go your way. If no one is available to teach you, you can always start your own discussions with your fellow peers in the same attachment.
- If you are corrected, do not take it personally. Instead, take it as a learning opportunity.

- You *will* *not* know everything. There will always be things that your preceptor knows but you do not know, even if you have prepared to impress.

As you step out into the acute settings, you will also begin to realise that many patients have other chronic diseases that need to be managed concurrently with their acute problem. Such diseases will be addressed in the chapter—Transition-to-Practice: Managing Chronic Diseases. You will also realise that being an RN is not a simple task, because it will never be just doing a single task. You need to be *sharp, observant, quick,* and *efficient* with *the ability to multi-task effectively.*

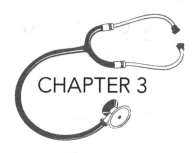

CHAPTER 3

NURSING MONITORING
AND MANAGEMENT

Besides carrying out the routine tasks and performing competent nursing skills, what are the other areas you need to know and possess to become an effective nurse? In this chapter, I will lay the foundations of the things you ought to know.

Vital Signs Monitoring and Common Critical Clinical Manifestations

Being able to take and interpret the vital signs of a patient is perhaps one of the most important and fundamental knowledge and skill as an RN. You need to know what is normal and what deviates from the normal. Monitoring and co-relating the vital signs to the patient's condition is essential to detect early deterioration of patient.

This chapter will include the four primary vital signs as well as conscious level and oxygen saturation to give a more wholesome view of the patient's condition in the ward. The four primary vital signs are body temperature, blood pressure, pulse rate, and respiration rate. In addition, the fifth vital sign, pain, will be included. The most common critical clinical manifestations in the ward will also be discussed to help you get more familiar and comfortable with working and learning the ward.

CONSCIOUS LEVEL

Glasgow Coma Scale (GCS)[2]		
Best Eye Response (E)	**Best Verbal Response (V)**	**Best Motor Response (M)**
4 Eyes opening spontaneously	**5** Orientated to time, place, person	**6** Obeys commands
3 Eyes opening to sound	**4** Confused	**5** Moves to localised pain
2 Eyes opening in response to pressure/pain	**3** Inappropriate words	**4** Normal flexion/ withdraws from pain
1 No response	**2** Incomprehensible sounds	**3** (Abnormal) flexion to pain
	1 No response	**2** Extension to pain
		1 No response

Table 1.2 Glasgow Coma Scale (GCS)

The GCS is a vital tool for assessing the patient's neurological status. It is usually embedded into the consciousness level chart (CLC). Monitoring for a decline in the GCS is important to minimise the potentially irreversible neurological damage to the patient. The maximum score is 15 while minimum score is 3 (*never zero!*). A patient's baseline GCS may not always be 15/15, hence, do not panic if you receive a patient with a baseline of less than 15. However, it is good to understand that there is *always* a reason for the patient's deviation from the best score. We should never assume that a deviated GCS

---

[2]   Graham Teasdale, "Forty Years on: Updating the Glasgow Coma Scale," *Nursing Times* 110, no. 42 (2014): 12–16.

is normal for any patient. Usually, a GCS drop of *two or more* from the baseline would be a great cause for concern. Vital signs should always be taken *in conjunction* with GCS decline to give a clearer picture of what is happening to the patient.

On conducting a GCS:

* Do make sure to understand the extent of patient's hearing/speech impairment, level of intellect (ability to understand simple questions), cultural/language differences, physical interventions (e.g., tracheostomy or sedative treatments), or existing deficits (e.g. hemiplegia) before conducting a GCS.

- Speaking close to patient's functional ear, call out patient's name.
- Assess for orientation/confusion using *"Time, Place, Person"*.
- While assessing the above, also look out for visual cues of understanding.
- Instruct the patient to do a finger squeeze on your finger. If eyes are closed and no response is present, you may induce pain by applying fingertip pressure, trapezius squeeze, or pressure on the supraorbital notch (listed in order of increasing discomfort).
- Your GCS score should be evident by now. Indicate 'NT' for sections not testable.

An extension to GCS is the CLC, which includes:

1. pupil size and reaction
2. limb movement

Pupil Size and Reaction[3]			
Eye (Left or Right)	Observation		
Pupil scale (mm)	1mm · 2mm • 3mm ● 4mm ● 5mm ● 6mm ● 7mm ● 8mm ●		
Pupil reaction to light	• Brisk • Sluggish • Fixed (No Reaction) • Not Tested (Eye Closed)		

Table 1.3 Pupil Size and Reaction[3]

Normal pupil size should range from 2mm to 4mm in bright light and 4mm to 8mm in the dark. Normal pupil reaction to light should be brisk. Dilated pupils with sluggish to fixed pupillary reaction to light may signify raised intracranial pressure (ICP). The clinical suspicion of raised ICP increases with unequal pupil sizes. On the other hand, pinpoint pupils may hint at opioid overdose, a possible condition for patients on high dose of narcotics for pain relief.

---

[3]   Ismalia De Sousa and Sue Woodward, "The Glasgow Coma Scale in adults: Doing it Right," *Emergency Nurse* 24, no. 8 (2016): 33–39.

> ### *On conducting a pupil size and reaction examination:*
> * Do ensure that patient is not on any eye drops that can cause the pupils to dilate or constrict as it will affect the accuracy of the test.
>
> - Measure and compare the pupil size of each eye.
> - Then, using a pen torch, shine from the outer canthus to the inner canthus of the eye.
> - Watch for constriction of the pupil and record observation.

Limb Movement[4]	
Type	**Description**
Normal	Overcomes gravity with maximum resistance.
Mild Weakness	Moves against gravity with mild to moderate resistance applied.
>Anti-gravity Strength	Able to lift a limb off the bed but unable to overcome resistance when applied.
<Anti-gravity Strength	Only able to move a limb along gravity plane. Not able to lift off the bed.
Minimal Strength	Demonstrates traces of muscle movement.
Absence of Movement	No motor strength.

Table 1.4 Limb Movement

Changes to limb power, especially when there are variations between the limbs may also demonstrate a neurological deficit or injury. Correlate findings in the CLC with vital signs to provide a clearer picture of the pathophysiology.

---

4   De Sousa and Woodward, "The Glasgow Coma Scale in adults," 33–39.

> ### On conducting a limb movement examination:
> * Do find out if patient has any previous stroke or other conditions that would affect the baseline of the limb movements before conducting the test.
>
> - Establish that the patient is able to obey commands.
> - Place one of your hands to each of the patient's upper or lower limbs.
> - Instruct the patient to resist your hands while you exert a downward force on:
>   i)   Palms of the patient's hands (upper limbs).
>   ii) The legs either near the ankle or knee (lower limbs).

In the next few pages, I will highlight a few conditions that commonly cause a decline in GCS +/- abnormal CLC in the acute setting.

Cerebrovascular Accident (CVA)

When a person is admitted to the ward with a medical or surgical problem, he/she might have other risk factors that predispose him/her to a CVA. Cardiovascular issues like *atrial fibrillation* (AF) puts the patient at a higher risk for a CVA. In AF, blood may not be completely pumped out of the heart. This may cause it to pool within the chamber of the heart and form a clot. This clot may become dislodged and then travels to the tiny blood vessels of the brain, obstructing blood flow to part of the brain which can result in an ischaemic stroke.

The risk of ischaemic stroke is also increased with *diabetes mellitus* (DM). When blood glucose levels are poorly controlled, it causes an increase in blood viscosity through a reduction in the deformability of the red cells. This causes an increase in their tendency to aggregate.

On the other hand, there are also patients who are more susceptible to haemorrhagic stroke. People who have a metallic heart valve, or heart conditions such as AF, may be on *anticoagulation therapy* (e.g. warfarin, rivaroxaban). Hence, their bleeding risk is higher than the average person. Poorly controlled hypertension also increases the risk of haemorrhagic stroke.

Understanding the risk factors as well as signs and symptoms of stroke will sharpen your clinical judgement for early detection and intervention to prevent irreversible damage to the brain or even death.

Immediate Management

Where CVA is suspected, RNs can use the FAST[5] method in conjunction with CLC/GCS to quickly judge whether a CVA is likely, to assist the medical team in planning for treatment and management.

F - Facial weakness/drooping
A - Arm weakness
S - Speech difficulty/slurred speech
T - Time to call a physician/Time duration

While consolidating findings from CLC/GCS, take vital signs STAT and inform the physician your suspicions immediately. Prepare patient for transport to radiology for an emergency CT brain/ CT angiography by bringing a **portable physiologic monitor** (+/- oxygen tank if needed) to continue monitoring patient's condition on the go. Be ready to also take blood profiles to help the physicians diagnose the type/cause of stroke and plan the appropriate treatment plan.

---

[5]   National Stroke Association, "Act FAST," accessed 12 March, 2018,
      http://www.stroke.org/understand-stroke/recognizing-stroke/act-fast.

Hypoglycaemia

A blood glucose level of less than 4.0mmol/L is known as *hypoglycaemia* and hospital protocols will require you to act even though many of the patients with diabetes tend to be asymptomatic. It is also a very common condition that is encountered in hospitalised patients, as their oral intake and appetite tends to be reduced in times of illness, thus it is **always** a good call to obtain patient's blood sugar levels (BSL) whenever there is a change in patient's mental status.

Reference range for random blood sugar levels[6,7,8]	
Low	< 4mmol/L
Normal	4-7.8mmol/L
Acceptable	7.8-11.1mmol/L
High	> 11.1mmol/L
Critical	> 33.3mmol/L (or "Hi" on glucometer)

Table 1.5 Reference Range for Random Blood Sugar Levels

There can be many reasons that contribute to hypoglycaemia, however, the most common two reasons encountered by a patient with diabetes in the hospital are listed below:

1. Alterations to appetite or oral intake and,
2. the administration of oral hypoglycaemic agent (OHGA) or insulin.

These factors are especially prominent in patients with diabetes because of the dependency on OHGA and synthetic insulin for blood glucose regulation. Continuing their regular dose of OHGAs or synthetic insulin *despite having a reduced oral intake* can bring the BSL to a dangerously low level.

Why is hypoglycaemia such a serious condition, especially when a patient is symptomatic? If you can recall in your pathophysiology, neurons are highly dependent on glucose for metabolism[9]. If this process is disrupted, it can lead to neuron dysfunction, coma, and even death very quickly. This shortage of glucose in the brain is known as *neuroglycopenia*.

Immediate Management

Watch for early signs of hypoglycaemia, such as giddiness, tremors, pale, cold and clammy skin. Late signs of hypoglycaemia would present with altered mental status/decreased GCS (confusion, drowsiness, unable to speak, seizures, or even unconsciousness). Check the BSL STAT once you suspect hypoglycaemia as a cause of the stated symptoms. Once hypoglycaemia is confirmed with the BSL reading, perform the following actions:

- Administer oral dextrose 15g drink if the patient is conscious.
- Recheck BSL 15mins later.
- Give another dose of oral dextrose if still hypoglycaemic.

An antidote for insulin (glucagon) may be required if the patient is not responsive to the dextrose drinks. If the patient is *drowsy* or *placed on nil-by-mouth order*, IV dextrose 50% will be needed to be given by the physician instead

---

[9]   Philipp Mergenthaler, Ute Lindauer, Gerald A. Dienel and Andreas Meisel, "Sugar for the Brain: The Role of Glucose in Physiological and Pathological Brain Function," *Trends in Neuroscience* 36, no. 10 (2013): 587–597.

(while waiting for the physician, RN may be allowed to give dextrose 20% infusion via a volumetric pump, depending on the hospital's policy).

Note: Please find out your hospital's protocol on hypoglycaemia management— the number of sachets of dextrose powder allowed to be administered and the interventions that an RN is allowed to do may vary.

Prevention

One of the best methods to prevent hypoglycaemia is through the **careful omission** of OHGAs and insulin when the patient is fasting, or have a very borderline BSL due to suboptimal appetite. Many patients in hospital may have reduced appetite and oral intake because they are unwell, not used to the hospital diet, or they may feel nauseous as a side effect of some medications. That is why monitoring and charting patients' meal intake can be helpful for the physicians in titrating DM medications.

Note: In some cases of poorly controlled DM, or in patients on total parenteral nutrition (TPN), they will still require their regular basal/long-acting insulin (e.g. isophane insulin) even while they are being kept nil-by-mouth.

BLOOD PRESSURE

Blood pressure (BP) is an indicator of haemodynamic stability. Systolic blood pressure measures the pressure on the vascular wall upon *contraction* of the heart, whereas diastolic blood pressure measures the pressure on the vascular wall upon *relaxation* of the heart. Variation of blood pressure can be a result of many conditions. To make things simple, I will only highlight problems that correlate with *extremely high and low blood pressures.*

✓ **Clinical Tips**
On taking blood pressure
* Do make sure to find out if there is a contraindication on any limbs (not to take BP on arm with an aterio-venous fistula (AVF) or on the side of previous mastectomy. Avoid swollen or injured limbs)

- Align artery marking on the BP cuff with the limb's artery, usually the brachial artery for arms.
- Make sure BP cuff is wrapped snugly. If forceful stretching is required or excessive free space is noticed, cuff size should be switched.
- Re-check BP using a manual BP machine if result fails to tally with clinical presentation or if there is a drastic difference from the previous reading.
- Do not attempt to increase BP by changing patient's position and chart the "improved" BP without understanding the cause.
- Take time to investigate the BP drop or increase and escalate the situation as necessary.

Hypertensive Crisis

Blood Pressure (BP) Categories	Systolic BP (mmHg)	Diastolic BP (mmHg)
Normal BP	< 130	< 85
High-normal BP	130–139	85–89
Grade 1 Hypertension	140–159	90–99
Grade 2 Hypertension	160–179	100–109
Grade 3 Hypertension (Hypertensive Crisis)	≥ 180	≥ 110

Table 1.6 Blood Pressure Categories[10]

10   Ministry of Health Singapore, *Hypertension: MOH Clinical Practice Guidelines 1/2017*, (Singapore, Ministry of Health Singapore, 2017), 18.

A systolic blood pressure (SBP) $\geqq$ 180mmhg or diastolic BP $\geqq$ 110mmhg is known as a *hypertensive crisis* because the pressure exerted by blood on the walls of blood vessels is potentially lethal. If the patient is *asymptomatic*, such elevation will be known as **hypertensive urgency**. A hypertensive crisis will present as a **hypertensive emergency** if the patient is *symptomatic* (i.e., evidence of organ damage). Micro-vessels, in particular, from the brain, eyes, heart, and kidneys cannot withstand such high pressures. Such an increase in pressure can cause giddiness (increased intracranial pressure), blurring of vision (swelling of the optic nerve), chest pain (myocardial ischaemia or infarct) and gross haematuria (rupture of glomerular capillaries). If vessels rupture in the brain, it will present as intracranial haemorrhage (ICH). Hence, there are potentially irreversible and life-threatening consequences to uncontrolled hypertension.

Immediate Management

In real world situations/hospital settings, you will see *a lot* of elevated BP in adult health. Some causes of elevated BP are not as urgent as compared to others. As an RN, you will need to know **when it is urgent or not**.

When the patient's BP is elevated (but <180mmhg), asymptomatic and close to their baseline, there is usually *no* urgent need to inform the physician, unless otherwise stated (e.g. if the patient has an aortic aneurysm, blood pressure control needs to be tighter and physicians may set the SBP limit at around <140mmhg[11]). BP can be also temporarily elevated after physiotherapy or when patients experience pain. Such issues will be expected to resolve with rest or with the relief of pain. You should watch for the return of BP back

---

[11]   Jade S. Hiramoto, Benjamin A. Howell, Linda M. Reilly and Timothy A. Chuter, "Effect of Systemic Blood Pressure on Aneurysm Size in the Presence of a Type II Endoleak," *Vascular* 16, no. 6 (2008): 321–325.

to baseline to confirm that the elevated BP is indeed due to transient triggers such as above.

However, when a patient is in a hypertensive crisis (≧180mmhg), whether symptomatic or not, the RN should inform the physician immediately (especially when the elevation is not related to pain or anxiety). Physicians should review the patient early if there is grade 3 hypertension, to determine if urgent treatments or investigations are required. Typically, if the patient is asymptomatic, oral antihypertensive will be given. If the patient is symptomatic, and/or there is a need to bring down the BP rapidly, IV antihypertensives may be given. The patient may even need to be prepared for transfer to High Dependency for closer monitoring.

Note: Do not treat the patient just by looking at the number. As a responsible nurse, **any raise in BP deserves a proper assessment** to establish whether it is required for escalation or increased frequency of monitoring.

Prevention

One of the best methods to prevent hypertensive crisis in an inpatient setting is the **prompt restarting** of oral antihypertensive drugs on admission, for patients with a background of hypertension, if this is not clinically contraindicated (e.g. patient is admitted for hypotension). If you notice that a patient has a known past medical history of hypertension, it is good practice to look through his list of medications to check if antihypertensives have been ordered up for him.

Hypotension

Maintaining sufficient blood pressure is essential as it concerns the adequacy of perfusion to vital organs. An SBP of *less than 90mmhg* would be a great cause for concern. Inadequate tissue perfusion would lead to cell death, organ damage and even organ failure. There are various types of shock, however, in the next section I will only cover two types of shock that are more commonly seen in the wards.

Hypovolaemic Shock (Progression of hypotension secondary to volume loss/blood loss)

The average adult has about 5L of blood, with a total volume of approximately 40L of fluid content (in an adult weighing 70KG). Patients who have undergone surgery can develop hypovolaemic shock due to loss of a large amount of body fluids. If bleeding is the specific cause of volume loss, it will be known as *haemorrhagic shock*.

Persistent vomiting, loose stools, extensive surface burns, or over-diuresis can also cause hypovolaemic shock to develop if no action is taken to replace what is lost. This is why monitoring of intake/output (I/O) is so important for certain patients. Do consider differences in body weight (patient with large body habitus is able to tolerate more volume loss than a smaller sized adult). Sometimes, the extent of volume loss may also not be obvious. For example, patients may pass only a small amount of per-rectal bleed or melaena, but there may actually be massive bleeding from the GI tract that has not yet passed out. Hence, attention should also be paid to vital signs and clinical signs – such as whether the patient is tachycardic and pale-looking.

Immediate Management

Along with I/O monitoring, vital signs monitoring would be required to detect the development and degree of shock. Remember, our body will always try to compensate in order to achieve haemostasis; RNs need to look out for signs and symptoms of compensation. *Initial haemodynamic compensation* includes tachypnoea then tachycardia. *Late signs of compensation* would present with hypotension, desaturation, then subsequently decline in GCS. It is essential that nurses detect and intervene at the earlier stages of compensation as it is easier to treat the patient as compared to the later stages where potential harm could have been done as well.

If IV fluid is administered rapidly (500mls over 15mins), this can increase the patient's BP. If profuse bleeding is suspected, an emergency blood transfusion would be warranted. In uncontrolled internal bleeding, an emergency procedure may be required to arrest the source of bleeding. IV tranexamic acid, an antifibrinolytic, may also be administered to stop bleeding. For visible external bleeding, such as from an open wound, pressure should be applied over the site of bleeding to achieve haemostasis. There may also be a need to close the bleeding point by suturing or cauterisation.

Note: Always be remindful of co-morbidities that patients have, such as renal and cardiac diseases, while giving a fluid challenge. Such patients are more easily susceptible to fluid overload or pulmonary oedema, which can present as breathlessness or low saturations.

*Additional Note: Reinforcing an already soaked dressing does **NOT** help in stopping the bleeding. Consider informing the physician to inspect the wound, as he may need to apply sutures, cauterisation, or even bring the patient to OT.*

Septic Shock (Progression of hypotension secondary to sepsis)

Patients may be admitted due to infections or develop infections during hospitalisation. These patients usually present with fever. Unfortunately, these infections can progress to sepsis and then to septic shock if antibiotic treatments are delayed or non-effective.

There are various factors influencing the success of treating the infections. They include:

- Source of infection (a brain abscess vs. a skin abscess)
- Identification of infection source(s)
- Promptness in the initiation of appropriate anti-infective treatment (microbiology culture and sensitivity results may take several days to be released)

- Co-morbidities (i.e. whether the patient is immunosuppressed, or has poorly controlled DM)

A *superficial* infection tends to be easier to treat as it can be quickly drained out through an incision or treated with topical antiseptics with lesser considerations. An infection that involves more delicate or deeper structures, like the liver, would require more scans and investigations before doctors decide whether to perform an invasive procedure, due to the greater risk of associated complications.

Sometimes, the complexity in the identification of the source of infection can cause delayed treatment. Furthermore, patients can develop new sources of infections during hospital stay (e.g. pressure sores, catheter-related infections, and hospital-acquired pneumonias) which can complicate things further.

Being able to detect the source of infection would be pertinent in rendering prompt and effective treatment. A physician can also decide to start on a broad-spectrum antibiotic treatment for the infection that he or she is suspecting, before a more definite microbiology report on specific culture and sensitivity is available, to prevent the patient's condition from deteriorating.

Immediate Management

Administer antibiotic treatment as soon as possible for the septic patient. Nurses should monitor for physical manifestations of worsening sepsis and compensatory mechanisms—like fever, tachycardia, and hypotension—as these may suggest that the patient requires escalation of antibiotics and/or the need for closer monitoring. It is also good practice to track the patient's progress after medical and surgical treatment has been rendered (e.g. evidence of scan showing reduction in the size of collections, downtrending inflammatory blood markers such as C-Reactive Protein (CRP), and total white cell count).

Nurses can sharpen their instincts at detecting possible *early deterioration* if they pay attention to patients' symptoms and behaviour while correlating with vital signs and laboratory results. This instinct helps nurses pre-empt their care and assists physicians in planning timely and effective treatments.

Additional Note: *To learn more about managing patient in deteriorating situations, do* **explore e-Rapids at https://courseware.nus.edu.sg/RAPIDS/e-simulation/ index.asp. It** *is a resource available for all to use.*

PULSE/HEART RATE

Normal resting heart rate is *between 60–100 beats per minute* (BPM). Variations to the heart rate can indicate an underlying disease process or pathology. For instance, if the patient is losing blood or going into a shock, the heart rate will increase to compensate for the loss of volume. Some of the common causes of abnormal increase in heart rate include:

- Hypovolemia (dehydration)
- Anaemia
- Infection/sepsis
- Pulmonary embolism

However, the heart rate can sometimes increase after the patient has consumed caffeinated products (like coffee, tea, or milo), after he/she has engaged in physical therapy, or even after venepuncture (which can be an anxious and stressful event for patients who are fearful of needles). In such cases, a repeated measurement after adequate rest is necessary to differentiate a temporary physiological response from an actual pathology.

In the same line of discussion, the heart rhythm can also tell us if the patient has any heart problems (e.g., heart block, atrial/ventricular fibrillation, or ischemia).

Supraventricular Tachycardia & Bradycardia

Supraventricular tachycardia (SVT) is when the heart beats so fast that it produces ineffective cardiac output because of decreased filling time. Hence, SVT produces symptoms of cardiac compromise. Typically, symptoms will only start appearing above 150bpm. On the other hand, symptoms of bradycardia usually manifest when HR<50. These conditions are more likely to be seen in a cardiac unit or telemetry ward. However, patients in the general ward may also develop such abnormal rhythms, especially in patients with existing cardiac issues.

General Management

In the general ward, when we detect a sudden significant increase or decrease in the baseline of the heart rate, or a new development of tachycardia or bradycardia, we should inform the physicians as soon as possible for investigations and corrective actions. There is *greater urgency* to inform physicians if clinical signs of cardiac compromise (with or without extreme heart rates) like palpitations, chest pain or tightness and SOB are present. The next step would be to help physicians find out the root cause, but at the same time, do not forget to monitor the rest of patient's vital signs and render supportive treatment as required.

The most common diagnostic at the ward level would be taking an electrocardiogram (ECG) and cardiac enzymes to rule out any cardiac events (3 sets over 24 hours may be required). Telemetry monitoring in the Cardiology ward or High Dependency Unit (HDU)/Intensive Care Unit (ICU) may be required. Management of abnormal heart rhythms should be in accordance with the Advanced Cardiac Life Support (ACLS) guidelines[12], where cardioversion, antiarrhythmic drugs, and/ or anticholinergic drugs may be administered. As the RN in-charge, you need to recognise the possible disease trajectory and standby for the crash cart, defibrillator, and the necessary IV drugs because every second matters to the patient's survivability in such fragile situations.

Additional note: Do a **manual palpation** of the radial pulse to check for pulse rate if you suspect that the recorded pulse rate does not correlate to the clinical presentation of the patient or if the recorded heart rate differs greatly from the patient's baseline.

RESPIRATORY RATE (RR) & OXYGEN SATURATION

Normal oxygen saturation is *above 95% on room air.* However, for patients with chronic obstructive pulmonary disease (COPD), their normal saturation may only be between 88% to 92% or higher depending on the severity of COPD. One of the greatest concerns about respiration is whether there is an increased effort in breathing manifested as shortness of breath (SOB).

Tachypnoea (increased respiration rate) indicates an *early compensatory mechanism* that the body is not able to achieve proper oxygenation. A decrease in oxygen saturation (spO2) is usually a later sign of poor oxygenation when the compensatory mechanism has started to fail. Thus, it is critical to alert the doctor early when a patient has an increased RR and manifests SOB, rather than waiting for a decreased spO2 (which is commonly practised in the wards). You should also investigate the possible underlying cause(s) of the increased RR while waiting for the arrival of the doctor and take early intervention to prevent further deterioration. It will be a relieving sight for the doctor when he/she arrives to see that you have already started the patient on supplemental oxygen with a working ECG machine

---

[12] ACLS Training Center, "Algorthims for Advanced Cardiac Support 2018," accessed 17 November 2018, https://www.acls.net/aclsalg.htm

on standby (and perhaps the radiographer is also alerted for a likely need of a portable CXR).

Common causes of abnormal increase in RR[13] include:

- Acid-base disturbances (acidosis versus alkalosis)
- Airway obstruction/constriction (e.g. asthma exacerbation)
- Pulmonary oedema (e.g. fluid overload)
- Chest infection (e.g. hospital-acquired/aspiration pneumonia)
- Psychological causes (e.g. pain and anxiety)

On the other hand, when the central nervous system is affected, bradypnoea (reduced respiration rate) can manifest. One of the most common presentations in the hospital is **opiate overdose** causing respiratory depression. In such cases, an opiate antidote (naloxone) would be required. Respiratory depression can also be a complication of a **traumatic head injury** and such trauma patients need to be closely monitored for late development of symptoms. Additionally, **obstructive sleep apnoea** is also increasingly commonly seen, especially in obese patients, and is a condition nurses should be trained to recognise as a respiratory risk.

When a sudden decrease of oxygen saturation occurs, and with other clinical manifestations, nurses need to be able to pre-empt certain events that may follow. Next, I will highlight the common conditions or situations where oxygen desaturation can happen in the ward.

---

[13]   Sheldon R. Braun, "Respiratory rate and pattern," in *Clinical Methods: The History, Physical, and Laboratory Examinations*, eds. Henry K. Walker, Wilbur D. Hall and John W. Hurst (Boston: Butterworths; 1990), chap. 43.

✓ **Clinical Tips**

On using the pulse oximeter

* Using the pulse oximeter on the same limb with the inflated BP cuff will cause a transient falsely lowered pulse rate and SPO2 due to blood supply being temporarily cut off when the BP cuff is being inflated.

- Avoid fingers with nail polish. Coloured polish that can absorb red light can lead to abnormal readings.
- Avoid shining bright light on pulse oximeter (operating theatre lights, heat lamps, sunlight).
- Avoid using on a limb with inflated BP cuff as it takes time for results to normalise.
- If extremities are cold (thus causing vasoconstriction), spO2 readings may not be accurate. Attempts at warming the fingers/toes may be helpful.
- Consider inaccuracy of reading in the presence of known carbon monoxide exposure or smoke inhalation from fire breakouts (most relevant in the emergency department setting).

Acute Respiratory Failure

Respiratory failure is a syndrome that arises from either one or both respiratory issues—hypoxemia and hypercapnia—causing the respiratory system to fail. Hypoxemia is inadequate oxygenation in the bloodstream, whereas hypercapnia is due to inadequate elimination of carbon dioxide from the bloodstream. Acute respiratory failure happens over a short period of time (hence patients are more likely to be symptomatic), whereas chronic respiratory failure occurs over a long period of time (hence patients may not always be symptomatic if they have developed some compensation). Here we will discuss some of the acute causes of respiratory failures.

Respiratory failure related to asthma/COPD exacerbation

Patients who have known history of asthma or COPD can develop acute exacerbation due to acquired infections, exposure to air pollutants and/or allergens, non-compliance to medications/therapies, and continued smoking.[14] The severity of exacerbations can vary, but the severe ones can lead to respiratory distress, failure and even arrest. When the inflammation processes set in, this causes swelling and bronchoconstriction, which limits the air entry into the alveoli for gas exchange.

Respiratory failure related to inactivity, aspiration or fluid overload (e.g. atelectasis, pneumonia)

Patients who have prolonged bed rest, are bed-bound or have persistent post-op pain are at risk of developing atelectasis. As their lungs do not expand to their fullest while they lie on bed for a prolonged period of time, (likewise for patients who fear taking deep breaths after operation due to pain), air sacs may fail to inflate properly. Fluid can accumulate and infection of the lungs may develop, causing SOB and respiratory distress.

Patients who have poor swallowing reflexes and inadequate gag or cough reflex have a high risk of developing aspiration pneumonia which subsequently leads to respiratory failure. In particular, stroke patients with swallowing deficits or elderly patients with functional decline are at increased risk of aspiration pneumonia.

Fluid overload is especially common in cardiac and renal patients due to reasons like over-hydration from IV medications and fluids, non-compliance to fluid restrictions, or a deterioration of their underlying medical condition. Fluid overload can cause pulmonary congestion and in severe cases, may require transfer to the ICU or High Dependency setting for ventilatory support.

---

[14] Stephen I. Rennard and Stephen G. Farmer, "Exacerbations and Progression in Disease in Asthma and Chronic Obstructive Pulmonary Disease," *Proceedings of the American Thoracic Journal* 1, no. 2 (2004): 70–92.

Respiratory failure secondary to circulatory issues (e.g. pulmonary embolism)

Patient with clotting disorders, deep tissue injuries, and/or prolonged bed rest can develop a thrombus in their veins—most classically in the veins of their lower limbs. The thrombus may be dislodged, then travels to the smaller vascular bed of the pulmonary vessels where it may become stuck. An ineffective gas exchange would then occur, which subsequently leads to respiratory failure if the clot is significantly large.

Note: Respiratory failure is the umbrella term for all the conditions causing ineffective air exchange between the lungs and blood. Do note that there are mainly two types (Type 1 and Type 2) of respiratory failures. Type 1—hypoxemia without hypercapnia. Type 2—hypoxemia with hypercapnia. Untreated respiratory failures can lead to respiratory arrest and subsequently death.

Immediate Management

Very often, *positioning* an alert patient to sit up improves ventilation for the patient and reduces the effort the patient requires to breathe. Propping the patient up is often easily done in the general ward setting.

The next immediate step is to *administer oxygen*. RNs should be familiar and confident with the standard oxygen supplementation tools—nasal cannula, simple face mask, Venturi mask, and non-rebreather mask.

Note: You can refer to the following guidelines of oxygen titration after the next page.

If you can hear gurgling noises or see secretions pooling around the patient's mouth, consider suctioning his/her oral cavity as these secretions may be causing airway obstruction. If the patient is nauseous or vomiting, consider placing him/her in a lateral position to avoid aspiration.

A patient with poor oxygen saturations can be assessed with a lung auscultation (yes, an RN should be able to do this) to determine the presence of lung sounds or any abnormal lung sounds (e.g. crepitus, wheezes, or rhonchi, etc.). This can help us identify respiratory problems early so that the relevant treatment can be initiated.

Diagnostic tests like arterial blood gas (ABG) results and CT pulmonary angiogram (CTPA) can help the medical team to find out the cause of inadequate oxygenation and increase efforts of breathing. As an RN, being able to anticipate these investigations can help you to be ready to assist and facilitate them.

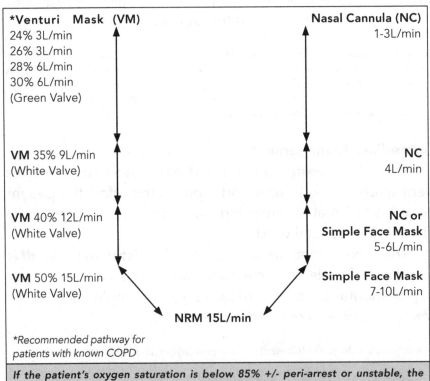

*Venturi Mask (VM)
24% 3L/min
26% 3L/min
28% 6L/min
30% 6L/min
(Green Valve)

Nasal Cannula (NC)
1-3L/min

VM 35% 9L/min
(White Valve)

NC
4L/min

VM 40% 12L/min
(White Valve)

NC or
Simple Face Mask
5-6L/min

VM 50% 15L/min
(White Valve)

Simple Face Mask
7-10L/min

NRM 15L/min

Recommended pathway for patients with known COPD

If the patient's oxygen saturation is below 85% +/- peri-arrest or unstable, the patient should be _immediately_ given 15L/min on NRM or bag the patient with (bag-valve-mask (BVM), even in patients with known COPD. Severe hypoxia can kill and needs to be rapidly reversed.

Table 1.7 Oxygen Titration[15]

15   BTS Emergency Oxygen Guideline Development Group, "BTS Guideline for Oxygen Use in Adults in Healthcare and Emergency Setting," *Thorax* 72, supp. 1 (2017): i1–i90.

Note: Allow at least 5 minutes for the oxygen saturation to stabilise before adjusting the next dose upwards or downwards for titration. The direct comparison between the FiO_2 of the Venturi mask and nasal cannula does not imply exact equivalence.

The Venturi mask is the only oxygen supportive device that is readily available in the general ward to allow *precise control* of the oxygen concentration. This can be very helpful for patients with known COPD, as high concentration of fraction of inspired oxygen (FiO_2) can actually reduce their hypoxic drive to ventilate. (The FiO_2 delivered by the Venturi mask is indicated by the percentage as shown in the *table above*.) However, in most acute cases, the respiratory symptoms that require escalation may be severe and a non-rebreather mask (NRM) is commonly needed to stabilise the patient. As a general guideline, it would be advisable to jump straight to administering NRM to a patient with spO_2 below 85%.

Care has to be undertaken when using a simple face mask. Using simple face masks with a flow of **less than 5L/min** can actually cause carbon dioxide rebreathing due to a build-up of carbon dioxide in the mask. This may worsen the oxygen saturation of the patient rather than helping them. The simple face mask is also known as a medium-concentration mask, which can deliver approximately up to **60% FiO_2**.

Many patients, however, would prefer to use nasal cannula due to its comfort and being able to speak while using it. The NC is also able to deliver medium-concentration oxygen therapy above 4L/min, but the higher flow rate may cause dryness to the nasal mucosa over prolonged periods of time. Consider using an *oxygen humidifier* for nasal cannula at higher flow rates, especially above 4L/min. Some institutions mandate compulsory humidifier for NC at 3L/min and above.

The drawback of the NC is that its FiO_2 cannot be accurately calculated due to varying breathing patterns of different patients. Do consider using an alternative to the NC for patients that are experiencing *SOB and/or breathing through their mouths.* Oxygen therapy through the NC are likely to be ineffective in such situations.

Should patients fail to respond to oxygen therapy through the above oxygen delivery appliances, non-invasive ventilation (NIV) may be used to support patient's breathing to prevent fatigue and improve oxygenation. If respiratory arrest is impending, invasive ventilation via intubation or an emergency tracheostomy may be necessary to secure the patient's airway.

Remember that if a patient either breathes too fast or too slow, or stops breathing, you can always assist and regulate the patient's breathing by forcing air in through a BVM.

Additional note: Do not underestimate the role of providing assurance to the patient who is hyperventilating due to anxiety and excessive pain.

Non-Invasive Ventilation (NIV)

There are two types of NIV system that can be used in a ward setting:

1. Continuous Positive Airway Pressure (CPAP).
2. Bi-level Positive Airway Pressure (BiPAP).

Common situations in which NIV are utilised are:

- Pulmonary oedema
- Obstructive sleep apnoea
- Respiratory failure
- Patients who are not candidates for intubation, i.e. limited by treatment status such as "Do Not Resuscitate" (DNR)

NIV is seldom used at the ward level routinely, especially because the support of respiratory therapists (RT) is needed to ensure that NIV is properly initiated. As nurses, our role in caring for patients with NIV would be to ensure the proper seal of NIV mask, the timely discontinuation and restarting of a set therapy, and to prevent pressure injury from prolonged use of NIV.

Patients may also bring to hospital their own NIV equipment when they are admitted—for instance, patients with sleep apnoea who are on long-term nocturnal CPAP. These devices, however, need to be checked each time they are admitted before being used in the ward. Typically, RTs should have *circuit breakers* for loan to prevent an event where the patient's CPAP device short-circuits the hospital's electrical supply. If patients on long-term CPAP therapy did not bring their devices with them to hospital, the hospital may have to loan out hospital sets of NIV for their usage.

Invasive Ventilation

There are two types of tubes used in invasive ventilation as described below:

- **Tracheostomy tube.** It is a tube inserted through a stoma made via an incision to the trachea from the neck. It comes in combinations of these *four variations:* cuffed or cuff-less, fenestrated or non-fenestrated. Fenestrated tubes are typically used while attempting to slowly wean the patient off a tracheostomy tube, or while trialling the use of a speaking valve. Tracheostomy tubes can be used for the long-term.
- **Endotracheal tube (ETT).** This tube is more commonly inserted from the mouth to the airway (orotracheal) than from nasal passage to the airway (nasotracheal). The tip of the ETT is placed at the carina, just before the bifurcation of the two main bronchi. An endotracheal tube is never used for the long-term, as the patient would need to remain unconscious (with or without anaesthesia) to suppress the gag reflex.

While patients are on invasive ventilation, it is important to monitor for patency of the airway. Secretions, with varying consistency and appearance, often interfere with the airway. These secretions can be as a result of local infection, bleeding, irritation, or the presence of a foreign object. Mucus plugging, a common complication with invasive ventilation, is a result of thick secretions/mucus forming a plug in the tube which can completely block off the airway. Monitoring and managing of secretions through humification and regular suctioning are essential in keeping the airway open. For patients with a tracheostomy, it is also necessary to standby a *tracheal dilator* at the bedside in order to keep the airway open in case the tracheostomy tube dislodges.

TEMPERATURE

Sepsis, an infective state where the patient is symptomatic with systematic inflammation response, is one of the leading causes of death in the hospital due to poor identification and delayed intervention. Despite fever being one of the important early signs of infection, there can also be a multitude of other reasons for causing variations in body temperature like age, individual person, activity, environmental temperature, consumption of hot food, time of the day, on-going infection, and omission of antipyretics. These factors may cause the temperature of a patient recovering in the hospital to go up to about 37.6° and slightly above, which alerts us that the patient is having a low-grade fever. However, typically, only when a patient's temperature exceeds 38.3°C,[16] the doctor may then want to take or repeat a blood culture **prior** to a new antibiotic treatment (if previously started on one) and do or repeat a septic workup.

---

[16]   David H. Bor, "Approach to the Adult with Fever of Unknown Origin," in *UpToDate*, ed. Ted W. Post (Walham: Massachusetts, 2018).

Note: If you initiate the empirical antibiotic therapy before the culture, there may not be enough causative bacteria that can be cultured and identified in the culture medium.[17] This may lead to inaccurate and less-directed treatment which can potentially cause more multi-drug resistant bacteria and poorer patient outcomes.

A septic workup usually includes:

- Culture and sensitivity (e.g. blood, urine, and/or samples from other suspected sources like wound, tissue, sputum, stool, and cerebral spinal fluid)
- Blood studies (e.g. full blood count, lactate, C-reactive protein, procalcitonin)
- Urinalysis
- Radiologic studies (chest X-ray and other scans for the suspected source of infection)

At this threshold, concerns of a new infective source or inadequate antibiotic cover would usually arise. However, this is not to say that below the temperature of 38.3°C would not require escalation, as bacteraemia can also exist even in the afebrile state or in low-grade fevers, especially in elderly patients and the immunocompromised, as their body's response to an infection may be blunted.[18]

Note: In the elderly population, the febrile response of the septic patient may be delayed and may not be the best marker to determine sepsis.[19] Therefore, it is always important to escalate not based on just one single vital sign, but collectively with your *assessment, clinical judgement, and reasoning.*

One of the biggest complaints from the doctors in the hospitals is the inability of nurses to appropriately communicate the need for review in a febrile or unwell patient. Sometimes,

---

[17]   Mitchell M. Levy and Andrew Rhodes, "The Surviving Sepsis Campaign Bundle: 2018 Update," *Critical Care Medicine* 48, no. 6 (2018): 997–1000.

[18]   Gary V. Doern, "Blood cultures for the detection of bacteremia," in *UpToDate*, ed. Ted W. Post (Walham: Massachusetts, 2018).

[19]   Prashant Nasa, Deven Juneja and Omender Singh, "Severe sepsis and septic shock in elderly: An overview," *World Journal of Critical Care Medicine* 1, no. 1 (2012): 23–30.

RNs may jump at a raised temperature reading and immediately call the physician for review, without being able to provide other relevant information such as—whether or not the fever is new, whether the patient is already on antibiotic treatment, and whether or not the patient's other vital signs and parameters are normal. Such calls can actually be *dangerous* to patient safety as they mask the calls that are urgent and needing physician review. Being able to communicative relevant information to the physician over the phone will help them determine how urgently they need to review this patient, especially if they have other tasks or patients to attend to. The RN is **not** simply a notification application that calls the physician for review whenever a reading is off, without critical thinking.

General Management

Wherever there is a raised temperature, the RN should perform a quick physical examination and review the trend of patient's vital signs, current available laboratory investigations and medications to assess the need and urgency for a doctor's review. A general guide for **escalation of antibiotic treatment or for medical re-evaluation** is when the patient is not showing signs of improvement or demonstrating progression of the degree of sepsis.

On a separate note, having a raised temperature can be distressing to the patient and patient's family as it is often accompanied with malaise. Hence, the RN should provide assurance to them, serve antipyretics where prescribed or allowed, and offer cold compress *regardless* of the need for medical review. The use of cold compress is very effective as a comforting measure if antipyretics cannot be administered.

✓ **Clinical Tips**

On using the tympanic ear probe

* Make sure patient's ear canal has no issues before inserting the ear probe (e.g. excessive ear wax, ear infection, or ear canal stenosis). Consider other forms of temperature-taking, such as using the axillary or rectal thermometer if you are doubtful of the accuracy of the measurement.

- Pull the auricle of the ear gently so as to straighten the ear canal.
- Insertion of the ear probe should then reach the desired position to accurately record the temperature.

PAIN

Being able to assess a patient's pain score accurately is important as pain can signal the presence of disease process and injury. Obtaining an accurate pain score is not an easy task, which can be more challenging if there are cultural or language barriers. However, there are several pain scale types that we can use to help us.

Types of pain scale commonly used:

- Numeric rating pain scale
- Verbal rating scale/simple descriptive pain intensity scale
- Wong-Baker FACES pain rating scale
- Behavioural pain scale

Note: Self-reported pain scale is the *gold standard* in pain assessment.

Each pain scale is suited to be used in different situations and patient profiles.

PAIN SCALE	PATIENT PROFILE OR SITUATION
Numeric Pain Rating Scale (NPRS)	Self-reported scale from 0 to 10 for all communicative and cognitively sound individuals.
Verbal Rating Scale/Simple Descriptive Pain Intensity Scale	Self-reported scale measuring intensity of pain, for all communicative individual who may not be able to fully appreciate the use of NPRS due to language barrier or inability to comprehend NPRS fully.
Wong-Baker FACES pain scale	Self-reported scale with pictorial guide designed originally for children aged 3 to 7, but it may be useful when there is a language barrier.
Behavioural Pain Scale	An observational scale scoring from 3 to 12, designed for mechanically ventilated patients but can also be used for patients with decreased consciousness.

Table 1.8 Pain Assessment[20]

General Management

There is always a tendency to reach out for the phone to ask the physician to order analgesia or just grab the medication cart to administer the analgesia whenever the patient complains of pain. However, it is also important to understand if the pain is related to the expected pathology of the patient's condition or indicative of greater severity. A bedside assessment should be performed to identify the likely cause of the pain. Otherwise, the way to manage pain can be guided by the World Health Organisation (WHO) analgesia ladder.

---

[20] Vertical Health, "List of Clinically Tested and Validated Pain Scales," accessed 19 November 2018, https://www.practicalpainmanagement.com/resource-centers/opioid-prescribing-monitoring/list-clinically-tested-validated-pain-scales.

Step-up if pain persists or increases

Step-up if pain persists or increases

Mild Pain	Moderate Pain	Severe Pain
Non-Opioids +/- Adjuvants	Weak-Opioids +/- Non-Opioids +/- Adjuvants	Strong-Opioids +/- Non-Opioids +/- Adjuvants

Non-Opioids: Paracetamol, Non-Steroidal Anti-inflammatory Drug (NSAID), Aspirin
Weak Opioids: Tramadol, Codeine, low-dose Morphine
Strong Opioids: Morphine, Fentanyl, Oxycodone
Adjuvants: Antispasmodic, muscle relaxant, corticosteroid, anticonvulsant, or antidepressant

Note: Combining drugs of different classes can increase the effectiveness of the analgesia, but not drugs of the same class.

Table 1.9 Pain Management[21]

The analgesia ladder was originally used to guide management of chronic cancer pain, but it has also been widely adopted as a guide to understand how to manage pain in general. It also teaches us how to administer analgesia more effectively.

21   World Health Organisation, "WHO's cancer pain ladder for adults," accessed 19 November 2018, http://www.who.int/cancer/palliative/painladder/en/.

✓ <u>**Clinical Tips**</u>
On pain assessment and pain management

- Always select a self-report pain scale over observational scale where possible, as pain is subjective. Pain is what the patient says it is.
- Manage the patient's expectation of pain and pain relief while serving analgesia as mismatched expectations may interfere with effective pain control. The patient's level of anxiety can contribute to more somatic symptoms and discomfort.
- Use your observational skills to guide your assessment on your patient's level of pain, and aim to match your objective assessment with the patient's report. For example, a patient may be frowning and perspiring, but he tells you that he has minimal pain as he fears taking more analgesia because of the possible side effects of the medication. In this case, perhaps what he needs is explanation and reassurance of how the analgesia works, so that he does not fear taking it when he is clearly in pain.

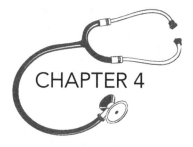

CHAPTER 4

NURSING KEY PERFORMANCE INDICATORS

The Ministry of Health (MOH) regularly reviews the incidences of hospital-acquired pressure ulcers and number of falls in hospitals to evaluate different institutions' practices and lapses in preventing such incidents. Thus, hospital management also pays a lot of attention to these two areas of nursing care as the institution may receive incentives or penalties, depending on the number of incidences.

Regular internal and external audits often take place within our healthcare institutions. As a nurse, your ability to perform some assessment and initiate intervention is critical. Often, the routine nursing task of two-hourly turning of immobile patients is ineffectively delivered if the nurse does not think critically to look beyond such routines. For example, patients who are continent are often placed on diapers in hospitals, especially if they have pain while ambulating and nurses wish to prevent falls in these "high fall-risk" patients. However, unnecessary use of diapers actually contradict with the measures of pressure ulcer prevention. In this situation, effective pain management may actually be the most critical intervention in preventing both pressure ulcers and falls during their hospitalisation. When we confine patients to the bed, not only do patients have high risk of pressure ulcer development, but they also have the potential of developing other complications like pneumonia, urinary tract infection, and physical deconditioning. We must acknowledge that *deconditioning* is also **harm** caused to the patient when we implement measures to confine their movements.

PRESSURE ULCER PREVENTION

Pressure ulcer is defined as an area of localised damage to the skin, muscle, and underlying tissue, caused by shear, friction, or unrelieved pressure, usually over bony prominences.[22] The use of Braden scale is recognised and widely used across the healthcare institutions locally. Having mastery of the scale would definitely benefit a nurse-in-training.

Braden Scale

The components of the Braden scale[23] are as follows:

- Sensory perceptions
- Moisture
- Activity
- Mobility
- Nutrition
- Friction and shear

The maximum score is 23 and the minimum score is 6. The *lower* the score, the *higher* the risk of developing pressure ulcer. As a guide, a Braden score of 15 and below would put a patient at risk of developing pressure ulcer. Scores of below 9

---

22   Ministry of Health Singapore, *Prediction and Prevention of Pressure Ulcers in Adults: MOH Nursing Clinical Practice Guidelines 1/2001* (Singapore: Ministry of Health Singapore, 2001), 1.

23   Nancy Bergstrom, Barbara J. Braden, Antoinette Laguzza and Victoria Holman, "The Braden Scale for Predicting Pressure Sore Risk," *Nursing Research* 36, no. 4, (1987), 205–210.

would put a patient at a *very* high risk. I will not break down the individual scores here as it is something very routinely done. However, I will discuss the different possible interventions for you to consider to prevent pressure ulcers from developing.

Some of the common nursing care for patients that are at risk of developing pressure ulcers include:

- **Initiate two-hourly turning.** Beneficial for patients who score low on activity and mobility, particularly, patients who are chair-bound to bed-bound.
- **Initiate air-mattress.** The effect is similar to turning the patient but it reduces pressure as a whole, in particular, at areas of bony prominence. This is necessary for patients with a particularly low overall Braden score. Poor nutrition weakens the skin and performing two-hourly turning alone may not be effective.
- **Cushion bony prominences.** Put up silicone (polyurethane) foam over areas of bony prominence. The sacrum tends to be more susceptible as it takes more effort to physically inspect this area.
- **Create moisture-barrier.** Consider using sting-free barrier spray (e.g. Brava®/Silesse/ 3M™ Cavilon™ No Sting Barrier Spray) over areas likely in contact with moisture or urinary/faecal matter. The spray creates a layer of protection on the skin so that the moisture will not weaken the skin. Use barrier cream (e.g. 3M™ Cavilon™ Durable barrier cream/ Conveen™ Critic barrier cream/SECURA◊ protective cream) for stronger protection, especially in denuded or macerated skin. Always apply creams *thinly*.
- **Do regular potting and diaper changes or put on urinary sheaths (for male patients).** Consider these if the skin contact time with waste matter is high due to factors like inability to move, verbalise needs, and eliminate urinary/faecal matter appropriately. Consider

the use of faecal diversions (e.g. Flexi-Seal™ SIGNAL™) for the patient with severe faecal incontinence.

- **Use slide/draw sheet to position patients on the bed.** This reduces friction and shear between the skin and bed-sheet, which can tear or erode the skin through physical mechanisms.
- **Start bed-cradle nursing.** This is for the badly macerated and eroded skin. Reducing moisture and moisture-contact through the removal of the diapers can be helpful for skin recovery and preventing further skin damage. Be mindful to maintain patients' privacy.
- Tailor nursing care with a combination of the above nursing interventions.

Much of the pressure ulcer prevention efforts are focused on relieving pressure/shear and reducing skin contact time with moisture/caustic fluids to prevent skin damage as a result of prolonged bed-rest. However, most of the time, the root cause of pressure ulcers is due to preventable issues like unnecessary diaper wearing and physical deconditioning due to over-zealous fall precautions, which result in patients having prolonged bed-rest. **Root causes** should always be addressed.

Remember, pressure ulcers *never* develop overnight. Make it a point to identify risks early and intervene whenever it comes to your knowledge. It takes a team to prevent pressure ulcers from developing.

FALL-RISK MANAGEMENT

A fall, as defined by the MOH nursing clinical practice guidelines, "is a sudden, unintentional change in position causing an individual to land at a lower level (either on an object or on the floor) other than as a consequence of sudden onset of paralysis, epileptic seizure or overwhelming external force".[24] The nursing role in the management of fall-risk includes thorough assessment coupled with the necessary interventions. One of the most common fall-risk assessment tools used in Singapore is the Morse fall scale.

Morse Fall Scale

The components of the assessment tool[25] include:

- History of falls
- Secondary diagnosis
- Ambulatory aids
- Intravenous therapy
- Gait/transferring
- Mental status

The maximum score would be 125 and the minimum score zero. A patient is at risk for fall when the score is 25 and above. A patient is at *high* fall-risk when it is 45 and above or as otherwise defined in your organisation. Each component carries a different scoring system.

The following interventions are as such:

- **Patient education.** Helping patients understand their fall risk and showing the available assistance for them (e.g. call bell) would definitely improve patient compliance to fall-risk precautions.
- **Environmental modifications.** Remove clutter and hazards (e.g. intertwined infusion pump wires, messy and misplaced cardiac tables) that might cause patients to trip. Ensure that bedrails are put up to help to keep patients in a safer environment.

---

24   Ministry of Health Singapore, *Prevention of Falls in Hospitals and Long Term Care Institutions: MOH Nursing Clinical Practice Guidelines 1/2005* (Singapore: Ministry of Health Singapore, 2005), 1.

25   Janice M. Morse, Robert M. Morse and Suzanne J. Tylko, "Development of a Scale to Identify the Fall-Prone Patient," *Canadian Journal of Aging* 8, no. 4 (1989): 366–377.

- **Adequate nursing attention.** Assist patients with IV drip during ambulation, use of commode for those who are unable to self-ambulate, and provide supervision for other ADLs as necessary.

- **Use of restraints.** This is the *last line* of intervention to be considered as it forcefully removes the patient's right to autonomy. Your institution should have guidelines on the application of restraints. In general, this should only be used when the patient's current condition poses as a threat to himself/herself or others around him/her.

- **Communication to the team.** Highlight patients with high fall-risk to the next shift and inform them what to look out for. Make sure fall-risk identification tags and signages are put up to help to alert anyone who is within the vicinity to be more vigilant.

- **Referral to the Physiotherapist.** Patients who are at risk of falling can be referred to the Physiotherapist for an initial assessment of their baseline level of function. This gives the multidisciplinary team a better gauge of the patient's level of function and allows them to take the necessary precautions or use the necessary gait aids to maximise safety and function at the same time.

With the above being said, the most essential trait of an effective nurse in preventing falls would be *vigilant eyes* and *acute awareness* of potential risks, while balancing it with respect for *the patient's autonomy and freedom of movement.*

Note: Do not confine the patient to bed just because of risk of falls. Forcefully putting up bedrails for restraint may increase the risk of falls and injuries.[26] Bedrails are designed as mobility aids and safety, not as a restraint. Consider 1-to1 nursing attention for the restless and cognitively impaired patient.

---

[26]   U.S. Food and Drug Administration, "Safety Concerns about Bedrails," last modified September 7, 2018, https://www.fda.gov/medicaldevices/products andmedicalprocedures/homehealthandconsumer/consumerproducts/ bedrailsafety/ucm362832.htm.

Deconditioning

Deconditioning is a process that involves physiological changes from sustained inactivity and bedrest. It can have a deleterious impact on well-being, especially in the hospitalised elderly. It has been associated with falls, functional decline, increased frailty and immobility, and predisposition to hospital-acquired pneumonia (HAP). All these contribute towards the patient's mortality and morbidity.

The hospital, with its natural imposed restrictions on activity, precipitates deconditioning. This happens especially when healthcare professionals are not watchful. Some of the reasons include:

CAUSE	EFFECT	
	PATIENT	NURSE
Organisational culture of blaming nurses for any falls involved	Reluctance to trouble nurses for activity due to line attachments (e.g. IV infusion, IDC), or maximum assistance required from staff.	Impose unnecessary activity restrictions (i.e. using diapers instead of encouraging mobilisation to toilet in continent patients) on patients due to fear of penalties when patients fall under their care.
Knowledge deficit on detrimental effects of prolonged bedrest/inactivity	Mentality that one should stay in bed until "fully recovered". Poor insight to own functional level/ weight-bearing status.	Does not appreciate his/her own role in preventing deconditioning. Unable to interpret PT/ OT assessment or input.

| Mobilisation & activity are **someone else's responsibilities** | Lack of self-motivation to participate in activity or therapy because of pain, tiredness, or disinterest. | Lack of proactiveness in getting review of mobility status (i.e. not taking initiative to suggest to physicians that a patient may benefit from PT/OT referral). |
| **Absence of advocates** for mobilisation/ No culture of pro-mobilisation | Reduced communication abilities (e.g. language barrier, speaking difficulties) | Mobilisation of patients not prioritised or seen as important for recovery. |

Table 1.10 Reasons for Prolonged Inactivity in Hospitals

Muscle atrophy has been found to occur as early as from **48 hours of bedrest**.[27] This means that patients should start moving as soon as they can or they should at least be engaging in some form of activity to reduce deconditioning. All healthcare professionals must begin to acknowledge deconditioning in hospitalised patients as harm, due to the downward spiral it can lead to.

---

[27]   Angela Gillis and Brenda Macdonald, "Deconditioning in the Hospitalized Elderly," *Canadian Nurse* 101, no. 6, (2005): 16–20.

- ↑ **Length of hospitalisation**
- ↑ **Risk of morbidity & mortality**

FEELING UNWELL/ MALAISE

RESULTS IN

- ↑ Functional Decline
- ↑ Frailty
- ↑ Immobility
- ↑ Risk of Falls & HAP

- ↑ Lethargy
- ↑ Reliance on others for ADLs

DECONDITIONING

PROLONGED BEDREST/INACTIVITY

- ↑ Muscle Atrophy
- ↓ Continence
- ↓ Independence in ADLS

Table 1.11 Vicious Cycle of Prolonged Inactivity

Prevention of Deconditioning

Nurses need to realise that the prevention of deconditioning in hospitalised patients is a *multidisciplinary effort* and everyone in the healthcare team has a part to play. Here are some simple steps that nurses can perform to decrease the possibility of deconditioning.

Patient Profile	Interventions			
• **Not allowed** to ambulate • Pre-morbidly **bedbound** (& able to follow commands)	• Bed Exercises • Sit up in bed	• Deep breathing exercises • Range of motion on bed/ chair (e.g. dorsiflexion/ plantarflexion of feet)		Obtain history and refer to PT/OT if patient is not at functional baseline
• **Allowed** to ambulate as tolerated • Pre-morbidly **wheelchair-bound** or **ambulant**	• Sit out of bed (SOOB) at meal times • Ambulation as per assessment			

Table 1.12 Simple Mobility Plan for Nurses

As a general rule, patients should not have bedrest unless indicated by team consensus for issues such as spinal fracture, post-angioplasty, or post-lumbar puncture. Even in critically-ill but stable patients in the ICU, patients are encouraged to do exercises such as deep breathing exercises or use an incentive spirometer. In the HDU, patients are also mobilised as tolerated with the help of a physiotherapist. In terms of ADLs, patients should be encouraged to undertake activities like wearing of hospital pyjamas, buttoning of clothing, and feeding as **independently** as much as possible. Nurses should play a greater role in advocating for maximising activity of hospitalised patients as part of their holistic care.

Functional Levels
Section co-written with **Matthew Neo Ji Hui**

Often as a nurse, you will refer to the physiotherapist's or occupational therapist's notes on the patient's pre-morbid (pre-admission) and current level of function. This will give you a good idea on how to aid the patient in their ADLs within the ward. Most physiotherapists (PTs) and occupational therapists (OTs) use standardised notations when documenting and it is worthwhile to be acquainted with their notations.

Functional Independence Measure[28]

The definition from this tool is most commonly used by PTs and OTs as a reflection of the amount of assistance that the patients need in their ADLs or functional activities such as ambulation, kerb crossing and stair climbing. PTs and OTs usually document each ADL or functional activity with their corresponding level of assistance to avoid confusion as a patient may be independent in getting out of bed but unable to stand due to severe foot pain.

---

[28]   John M. Linacre, Allen W. Heinemann, Benjamin D. Wright, Carl V. Granger and Byron B. Hamilton, "The Structure and Stability of the Functional Independence Measure," *Archives of Physical Medicine and Rehabilitation* 75, no. 2, (1994): 127–132.

ASSIST LEVEL	WRITTEN AS	DEFINITION	
Complete Independence	I	All tasks are performed safely without modification, assistive devices or aids and within reasonable time with no assistance required. The patient is able to perform the activity safely alone.	NO HELPER REQUIRED
Modified Independence	Mod. I	One or more of the following are true about the activity: • requires an assistive device • takes more than reasonable time • there are safety (risk) concerns Still, no manual assistance or helper required.	
• Stand by Assistance • Supervision or Set-up	SBA or S/V	Requires no more than standby, cueing or coaxing without physical contact or helper sets up needed items or applies orthoses.	
Contact Guard Assistance	CGA	Variation of minimal contact assist where subject requires contact to maintain balance or dynamic stability.	

Minimal Contact Assistance or Minimal Assistance	Min contact A or Min A	Requires no more than touching & expends 75+% or more of the subject's effort; assistance is needed to lift one limb.	
Moderate Assistance	Mod A	Requires more help than touching or expends 51% to 75% of the subject's effort; assistance is needed to lift two limbs.	HELPER REQUIRED
Maximal Assistance	Max A	Subject expends only 26% to 50% of effort.	
Total Assistance	Total A	Subject expends less than 25% of effort; two or more helpers required for assistance.	

Table 1.13 Functional Independence Measure

While most PTs and OTs do try to follow this standard of documentation, nonetheless there will always be some deviations. For example, a notation of "Max A x 2" essentially means that the patient requires total assistance from two helpers. Why "Max A x 2" is documented may be a result of "total assistance" being a notation not commonly used in the local context.

Another caveat here: as with any assessment, is that they usually only hold true at the point of assessment. For example, if the patient falls further ill during their stay, it would only be reasonable to say that previous assessments by the PTs and OTs may not be valid. Thus, it is good to check with the patient's respective PT and OT on the most updated functional status.

Finally, the assessment usually includes the type of gait aid that the patient uses. Hence a CGA with w/f (Contact Guard Assist with Walking Frame) would signify that the patient requires a walking frame to achieve a contact guard level of assistance.

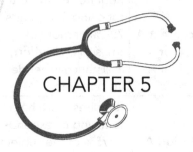

CHAPTER 5

ACTIVITY TOLERANCE/ RESTRICTION STATUS

While physical activity is good in general, some patients need to have activity restrictions placed on them to aid in their recovery or to prevent further injuries.

Complete Rest in Bed (CRIB)
This is a status that is common for patients who underwent angioplasty (be it on the limb or heart). Patients are required to lie flat in bed for *six hours* to prevent bleeding or formation of haematoma at the incision site. A CRIB status may also be in force when acute myocardial infarction or hip fractures are suspected. If a fracture of the spine is suspected, spinal nursing would be necessary.

Rest in Bed (RIB)
Patients are allowed to move in bed (i.e. turning) with the head of bed elevated. They are not allowed to transfer out of bed because transferring and ambulation can be too strenuous for them. Such activities can increase blood pressure or worsen cardiac conditions that may be dangerous for certain groups of patients.

One such group of patients are those with aortic aneurysm or aortic dissection. Typically, the goal would be to keep their SBP less than 140mmhg. Ensuring a good BP control for such a group of patients would then be important before ambulating or escalating activity tolerance.

It is worthwhile to note that CRIB and RIB may be used interchangeably in the local context, hence corroborating the status with the documentation would be sensible.

Sit out of Bed (SOOB)

Patients who have undergone surgical operations may have prolonged bed rest due to pain, fear of pain, and fatigue. *Older patients* tend to decondition more after prolonged bed rest. These groups of patients should be encouraged, at the earliest opportunity, to SOOB and have SOOB regimens (e.g. SOOB (TDS)) assisted by the staff nurse or PT/OT. SOOB can reduce the chances of developing pneumonia, atelectasis, and deep vein thrombosis. Patients who SOOB as soon as they are medically stable to do so, tend to look and perform better during the recovery period, from my observation in my practice and supported by research.[29]

Encourage ambulation as tolerated

Patients who are stable medically are encouraged to ambulate as much as they can. However, some patients may have difficulty to move around because of bodily modifications (e.g. amputations, fractures), improper techniques while attempting to adapt to body modifications, or pain on movement after surgery. Also, they may not be suitable for

---

[29]   Barbara Liu, Julia E. Moore, Ummukulthum Almaawiy, Chan Wai-Hin, Sobia Khan, Joycelyne Ewusie, Jemila S. Hamid, Sharon E. Straus and MOVE ON Collaboration, "Outcomes of Mobilisation of Vulnerable Elders in Ontario (MOVE ON): a Multisite Interrupted Time Series Evaluation of an Implementation Intervention to Increase Patient Mobilisation," *Age and ageing* 47, no. 1, (2017): 112–119.

putting the full pressure of their body on a particular limb with fractures or surgical fixations. In such circumstances, the physicians would then suggest a *partial* weight-bearing status or a modified partial weight-bearing status (e.g. heel, toe-touch) for ambulation.

DEFINITIONS OF WEIGHT BEARING STATUSES
*Section co-written with **Matthew Neo Ji Hui***

TERM	DEFINITION
Non-Weight-Bearing (NWB)	The leg must not touch the floor and is **not** permitted to support any weight at all. 0% of body weight to rest on leg. The patient usually uses crutches or a gait aid to hop on the other leg but this depends on the patient's level of comfort in doing so. Elderly patients may not take to ambulating with an NWB status on one foot.
Touch-Down Weight-Bearing (TDWB) or Toe-Touch Weight Bearing (TTWB/TWB)	The foot or toes may touch the floor (such as to maintain balance). Most doctors allow up to 10% of body weight to be placed on the foot.
Heel Weight Bearing (HWB)	The heel can support the weight of the body. Usually seen in patients undergoing toe amputations. The podiatrist may prescribe special shoes to improve the patient's comfort level.
Partial Weight Bearing (PWB)	A small amount of weight may be supported by the affected leg. The weight may be gradually increased up to 50% of the body weight. Gait aids are still mandatory. Single sticks are not allowed.
Weight Bearing as Tolerated (WBAT)	Patient is allowed as much weight as they feel comfortable with. Gait aid use is at the discretion of the treating physiotherapist.

Protected Weight Bearing (PTWB)	Weight bearing as tolerated but gait aids are mandatory at all times until further follow-up with the surgeon.
Full Weight Bearing	100% of body weight on leg. Walking without an aid is allowed.

Table 1.14 Weight Bearing Statuses

You will often also see that a patient may have more than one weight bearing status. For example, after a road traffic accident (RTA) and sustaining multiple fractures and injuries, a patient may be NWB on the right upper limb, PWB on the left lower limb, FWB on the left upper limb and WBAT on the right lower limb. With so many different weight bearing statuses, you may find it overwhelming at first. However, there is no need to worry as the attending PTs and OTs will assess the patient to try out different methods of ambulation or moving about which you can observe and learn from.

PTs play an important role in teaching and motivating the patients to adapt to new techniques for ambulation. They will also prescribe strengthening exercises for patients to maintain their muscle mass or respiratory health while in the hospital.

OTs help patients overcome their deficits by teaching them techniques for them to continue doing their ADL. Some examples include buttoning with one hand, introducing an adaptive aid for scooping up food for the hand that lost its dexterity, or transferring oneself safely to the wheelchair using one leg.

Nurses play a *pivotal role* in motivating patients to engage in therapy as rehabilitation aids in recovery. By discussing with the therapists, nurses can aid in reinforcing and encouraging activities like deep breathing, bed exercises, and ambulation even after office hours when the therapists are not around. The hospital setting as well as most patients' initial mindset result in them staying in bed for nearly the whole day while awaiting treatment to be rendered. Unless absolutely necessary, resting in bed the whole day has been proven to be detrimental to respiratory and musculoskeletal health.[30] Hence, keeping patients active and optimising their function become a shared responsibility of the entire team.

---

[30]   Selina M. Parry and Zudin A. Puthucheary, "The Impact of Extended Bed Rest on the Musculoskeletal System in the Critical Care Environment," *Extreme Physiology & Medicine* 4, no. 16, (2015): doi:10.1186/s13728-015-0036-7

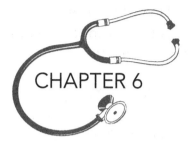

CHAPTER 6

DIETARY MODIFICATIONS & RESTRICTIONS

Knowing and understanding the dietary restrictions for your patients is important because you will need to be able to explain to patients why they are put on certain restrictions. There is much truth to the classic statement, *"a hungry man is an angry man"*. Pay attention to this and you can avoid a lot of potential troubles.

Nil-by-Mouth (NBM)

Fasting can be a part of surgical preparation, but it could also be a treatment due to recent interventions that have been done to the digestive system. Surgeries done to the stomach, small and large intestines, pancreas, and the gallbladder can modify the patient's diet requirements drastically.

Indications for NBM include:

- Pre-operative preparation
- Post-operative rest of the gastrointestinal (GI) tract (e.g. to protect anastomoses)
- GI tract problems (e.g. obstruction, motility issues)
- Unsafe for oral feeding (e.g. decreased consciousness, dysphagia, persistent nausea and vomiting)

When patients need to go through general anaesthesia (GA), they just need to fast for at *least two hours for liquids* and *six hours*[31] *for solids* to prevent aspiration, as recommended by various anaesthesia societies.

Note: Most of the time, patients tend to over-fast due to standard orders of "NBM from 12 midnight", even though surgeries may not be performed first thing in the morning. As a nurse, you should advocate for minimal fasting time to improve the patient's experience of going for a surgery.

Furthermore, as an RN, you can also place patients on NBM if you have reasons to believe that the patient is unsafe to eat per orally. Subsequently, discuss possible referrals (e.g. to Speech Therapist) and other interventions (e.g. NGT insertion for decompression) with your physicians for safe feeding or appropriate dietary restrictions. Also, remember that diabetic patients who are kept NBM should usually be on a dextrose-containing drip (refer to your hospital policy) to prevent hypoglycaemia. It is important to have proper and early education when patients are kept fasted, as it promotes patient compliance and rapport between patient and nurse.

DIET & FLUID MODIFICATIONS
Section co-written with **Janice Tang Si Jia**

Diet and fluid modifications are introduced for patients with deficits in their ability to swallow or manipulate food. Swallowing difficulties are termed as dysphagia. The Speech Therapist (ST) will assess the patient to determine the severity and impact of the dysphagia before recommending specific diet/texture consistencies suitable for the patient to consume safely.

Diet/fluid modifications are based on the International Dysphagia Diet Standardisation Initiative (IDDSI).

---

[31]   Christopher J. Jankowski, "Preparing the Patient for Enhanced Recovery After Surgery," *International Anesthesiology Clinics* 55, no. 4, (2017): 12–20.

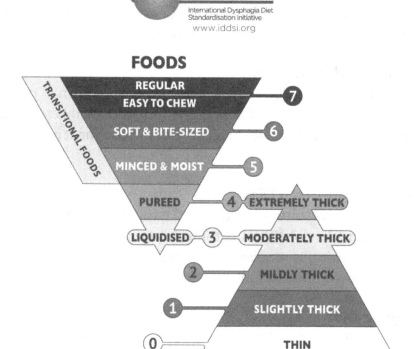

Figure 1: IDDSI Framework[32]

Puréed Diet

This is usually for patients with permanent impairment or deficits in their ability to swallow. It contains all the nutrition of a normal meal (i.e. with meat and vegetables but blended into a smooth texture of *no lumps*). Puréed diet holds its shape on a spoon and falls off easily if the spoon is tilted. Example of puréed foods include mashed potato and yam paste.

However, a lot of patients have initial problems adapting to this diet because the enjoyment of eating is diminished and

---

[32] International Dysphagia Diet Standardisation Initiative, "IDDSI Framework," last modified March 31, 2019, https://iddsi.org/framework/.

the taste may be altered. Hence, it is often the last resort if swallowing rehabilitation is limited.

Otherwise, tube feeding would be recommended if there is a risk in aspiration or if silent aspiration cannot be ruled out.

Minced and Moist Diet

Minced diet is very soft and is cut into very small moist lumps of 0.4cm. *Minimal chewing* is required for this texture. An example of minced texture includes minced meat or cut-up 'chai tow kway'.

Soft and Bite-Sized Diet

Food that is softer in texture and easier to digest. Soft diet is also tender, moist, and cut into bite sizes, no bigger than 1.5cm. Chewing is required. Examples of soft diet are cut-up banana, 'chee cheong fun', and cake.

Regular Diet

No medical problems exists to warrant any restrictions on diet. It is normal that everyday foods of various textures need biting and chewing abilities. Examples of a regular diet includes biscuits, fried foods, and noodle soup.

Normal everyday foods of soft/tender textures with no restrictions to food particle size are called "Easy to Chew". Examples include steamed fish and scrambled eggs.

Other Restrictions

Patients with suspected swallowing impairments should be assessed by the ST. The most common reason for referral by nurses is coughing or choking while attempting to swallow. After the assessment, the ST would decide which consistency is the best for the patient to consume his/her food safely. They may recommend the use of food thickener, or recommend a particular way of eating food or drinking fluids (e.g. tablespoon feeding or cup feeding).

Food Thickener

The use of a food thickener is to change the consistency of a particular fluid to one of the following thickness:

- Slightly Thick (thicker than water)
- Mildly Thick (similar to texture of cough syrup, cream soup and base of barley water)
- Moderately Thick (similar to texture of yogurt and smoothies)
- Extremely Thick (similar to texture of mousse)

Different brands of thickeners may have varying methods for thickening, so do speak with your ST to find out the method of preparation when in doubt. By altering the fluid consistency and modifying the feeding technique, the patient would be able to swallow with significant reduction in aspiration.

Note: Current evidence for the role of food thickener in reduction of aspiration pneumonia is mixed due to decreased satiety and increased dehydration, causing worsening of dysphagia.[33] In fact, there is stronger evidence that maintaining good oral hygiene may be more important than fluid consistency modification in preventing aspiration pneumonia.

Additional Note: Always sit patient upright as much as possible when they are having diet to prevent aspiration (including patients on naso-gastric feeding). 90° upright would be the most ideal position.

DIETARY RESTRICTIONS
Section co-written with **Hoong Jian Ming**

Clear Feeds

This is a gentle diet consisting of only *clear* liquids. It is to put the patient on trial for tolerance of diet +/- post-operatively/post-scopes, or for patients recovering from GI

---

[33]   Tay Wei-Yi, Low Lian-Leng, Tan Shu-Yun and Farhad F. Vasanwala, "Evidence-based Measures for Preventing Aspiration Pneumonia in Patients with Dysphagia," *Proceedings of Singapore Healthcare* 23, no. 2, (2014): 158–165.

tract problems such as partial GI obstruction, GI bleed, and/or paralytic ileus. It should be easily digested and leaves no residue in the gastrointestinal tract. Drinks can be considered as a clear liquid if you are **able to see through it.** Examples of clear liquids include plain water, coffee/tea without milk, clear fruit juice, clear jelly, cordials, and juice-based nutrition supplements.

Full Feeds

This is an escalation of diet from clear feeds before transiting to soft diet or diet of choice (DOC). Examples of full feeds include milk, soy milk, strained juices, plain pudding, ice cream, coffee/tea with milk, creamed soup, and milk-based nutrition supplements.

Note: Liquid diets are usually inadequate to meet patient's nutrition needs. Normally, it should not be used for more than a few days. Do check with the medical team or the Dietitian if there is a need to initiate enteral/parenteral feeding if your patient is persistently kept on a liquid diet.

Diet of Choice (DOC)

There is no dietary restriction. However, do take note if there are any texture or fluid modifications recommended by the Speech Therapist or medical team.

Diabetes Mellitus (DM) Diet

This is catered to DM patients and aims to avoid post-prandial spikes in blood sugar levels. The carbohydrates throughout the day are evenly distributed according to nutritional requirements. The diet is also low in sugar and fats and high in fibre.

Low Residue/Fibre Diet

Low residue diet is given for bowel rest and is frequently utilised for patients who have gone through bowel resections and those experiencing bowel flares. It is also for patients who require bowel preparation the night before colonoscopy. It is useful as it reduces bulky stool formation with less mechanical bowel movement.[34] This diet is also recommended for patients after the creation of an ostomy to reduce the possibility of a bowel obstruction.

A low residue diet is usually prescribed by the medical team for pre-colonoscopy bowel preparation or for the management of gastrointestinal conditions such as inflammatory bowel disease (IBD).

The European Society of Gastrointestinal Endoscopy (ESGE) recommends a low-fibre diet on the day preceding colonoscopy but does not make any recommendations regarding the use of low-fibre diet for more than 24 hours prior to the examination.[35]

Prolonged use of low residue diet for acute IBD or IBD in remission is discouraged due to the lack of evidence for such restrictions.[36] For post-operative bowel recovery, it theoretically reduces bulky stool formation hence decreases bowel activities, allowing bowel rest. It also reduces the possibility of a bowel obstruction. However, there are also limited evidences for such practice. The ERAS protocol increasingly recommends a diet of choice within 24H post-operatively.[37]

---

[34] Wu Keng-Liang, Christopher K. Rayner, Chuah Seng-Kee, Chiu King-Wah, Bruce Lu and Chiu Yi-Chun, "Impact of Low-Residual Diet on Bowel Preparation for Colonscopy," *Diseases of the Colon & Rectum* 54, no. 1, (2011): 107–112.

[35] Cesare Hassan, Michael Bretthauer, Michal F. Kaminski, Marcin Pólkowski, Björn J. Rembacken, Brian Saunders, Robert Benamouzig, Oyvind Holme, Susi Green, Teaco Kuiper, Raccardo Marmo, Mohamarowi Omar, Lucio Petruzziello, Cristiano Spada, Alberto Zullo and Jean M. Dumonceau, "Bowel Preparation for Colonoscopy: European Society of Gastrointestinal Endoscopy (ESGE) Guideline," *Endoscopy* 45, no. 2, (2013): 142–155.

[36] Natasha Haskey and Deanna L. Gibson, "An Examination of Diet for the Maintenance of Remission in Inflammatory Bowel Disease," *Nutrients* 9, no. 3, (2017): 259.

[37] Joseph C. Carmichael, Deborah S. Keller, Gabriele Baldini, Liliana Bordeianou, Eric Weiss, Lawrence Lee, Marylise Boutros, James McClane, Liane S. Feldman and Scott R. Steele, "Clinical Practice Guidelines for Enhanced Recovery After Colon and Rectal Surgery From the American Society of Colon and Rectal Surgeons and Society of

A 'low residue diet' and 'low fibre diet' are technically different but are often incorrectly used interchangeably; however, we shall leave this discussion to another day.

Low Salt (Sodium) Diet

This diet is prescribed for patients with certain chronic conditions such as hypertension, chronic kidney disease, heart failure, and liver failure with ascites. The saying, "where sodium goes, water follows", is pertinent to patients with problems getting rid of water in their body as increased salt intake would work against water expulsion from the body. This diet limits the amount of sodium in the diet. It limits food such as gravy, processed food, added sauces, and condiments in the diet. In hospitals, the food service usually works with the Dietitian to standardise recipes to ensure that the ingredients used and food served are low in sodium.

Low Fat Diet

This diet is prescribed for patients who need to restrict their fat intake, including patients who need to lose weight, patients with cardiovascular risk factors such as hyperlipidaemia and diabetes, or patients who have fat maldigestion or malabsorption (e.g. diseases of the gallbladder or pancreas).

Note: Some patients on diet restrictions may ask for "tastier" meals. Understanding the role of "low salt" and "low-fat" diets can help you address some of the patients' commonly asked questions.

Low Potassium, Low Phosphate Diet

This diet is prescribed for patients with renal impairment or failure. In patients with renal issues, hyperkalaemia and hyperphosphataemia can develop due to the kidney's inability to excrete certain electrolytes. Hence, food with higher contents of potassium and phosphate should generally be

American Gastrointestinal and Endoscopic Surgeons," *Diseases of the Colon & Rectum* 60, no. 8, (2017): 761–784.

avoided. Phosphate-binders such as calcium acetate tablets are also commonly served pre-meal, to bind with phosphate in the gastrointestinal tract, making it unavailable to the body for absorption.

Note: Common snacks such as Milo and wheat biscuits can be high in phosphate. Do check with your institution's foodservice to determine what snacks are available for patients who require such restrictions.

NUTRITION SCREENING
Section co-written with **Hoong Jian Ming**

Malnutrition is common in a hospital setting and is associated with poor clinical outcomes, including functional decline, poorer wound healing, increased length of hospital stay, and increased mortality. Despite such negative outcomes, malnutrition is often *not identified*, possibly due to its slow and insidious effect. Hence, nurses play an important role as patient's advocates to carry out nutrition screening in order to facilitate assessment and identify malnourished patients for timely nutritional interventions.

Each institution should have protocols in place to systematically screen patients for malnutrition on admission using a nutrition screening tool. Examples of nutrition screening tools are the Malnutrition Universal Screening Tool (MUST)[38], Malnutrition Screening Tool (MST)[39], Nutritional Risk Screening (NRS 2002)[40], 3-minute Nutrition Screening Tool (3-MinNS

---

[38] Marinos Elia, *The 'MUST' Report* (The British Association for Parenteral and Enteral Nutrition, 2013): 1–127.

[39] Maree Ferguson, Sandra Capra, Judy Bauer and Merrilyn Banks, "Development of a Valid and Reliable Malnutrition Screening Tool for Adult Acute Hospital Patients," *Nutrition* 15, no. 6 (1999): 458–464.

[40] Jens Kondrup, Henrik H. Rasmussen, Ole Hamberg, Zeno Stanga and Ad Hoc ESPEN Working Group, "Nutritional Risk Screening (NRS 2002): A New Method Based on an Analysis of Controlled Clinic Trials," *Clinical Nutrition* 22, no. 3 (2003): 321–336.

Tool)[41] and Mini Nutritional Assessment (MNA®)[42]. Do check with your institution on the tool that is used in your hospital. These tools are easily accessible on the internet.

Most screening tools utilize similar measures to determine nutrition risk:

- **BMI**: This can be obtained using the equation: $\frac{weight\ in\ kg}{(height\ in\ m)^2}$
- **Weight**: This can be obtained using a stadiometer, weighing chair/bed, or even by asking the patients or their family members. Do check the date when the weight was taken if it is obtained from the electronic health records.
- **Weight History**: This can be obtained from the patients, their family members or from electronic medical records. Some tools will require you to calculate a percentage weight loss over a period of time. Use the formula: $\frac{previous\ weight\ -\ current\ weight}{previous\ weight} \times 100\%$ to obtain a percentage of weight loss/gain.
- **Oral Intake**: This can be obtained from the patients or their caregivers and family members. You can ask if the patient had a reduced dietary intake in the previous week, followed by how many percent lesser than the usual portion he/she is taking if there is a reduced dietary intake.
- **Physical Assessment**: If the tool requires the use of a physical assessment, in-service training should be provided by the institution to identify muscle wastage.
- Other measures such as mobility, psychology stress, acute illness may be required but these are all fairly

---

[41] Lim Su-Lin, Tong Chung-Yan, Emily Ang, Evan Lee, Loke Wai-Chong, Chen Yu-Ming, Maree Ferguson and Lynne Daniels, "Development and Validation of 3-Minute Nutrition Screening (3-MinNS) Tool for Acute Hospital Patients in Singapore," *Asia Pacific Journal of Clinical Nutrition* 18, no. 3 (2009): 395–403.

[42] Yves Guigoz, Bruno Vellas and Philip J. Garry, "Assessing the Nutrition Status of the Elderly: The Mini Nutritional Assessment as Part of the Geriatric Evaluation," *Nutrition Reviews* 54, no. 1 (1996): S59–S65.

straightforward information that can be obtained from the patient or their caregivers or family members.

The nutrition screening tool will generate a score at the end of the screening, which will correspond to a follow-up action. This action can range from ongoing monitoring and a rescreen after a period of time, to a referral to a dietitian for further in-depth nutrition assessment. For example, the 3-MinNS Tool recommends a referral to the dietitian if the score exceeds 3. The MUST recommends a rescreen every week for hospitalised patients whose score is at 0 (low risk); the documentation of dietary intake for three days and then take necessary follow-up actions if the score is 1 (medium risk); or a referral to Dietitian or Nutrition Support Team if the screening score is 3 (high risk). Hence, nutrition screening serves as an important window of opportunity to identify patient at risk of malnutrition. Nurses in the wards can help this process by conscientiously screening all patients on admission.

Management of Malnutrition

As mentioned earlier, following nutritional screening, there will be some corresponding actions to be done. Here is a simple management plan to help nurses internalise the approach towards patients at risk of malnutrition.

LOW–MEDIUM RISK	HIGH RISK
Patients with alterations to their oral intake due to illness or fasting. Predicted period of alteration is short and likely resolvable.	If patient is acutely ill **and** there has been/predicted to have little or no nutritional intake for >5 days.

Observe	**Treat**
• Watch dietary intake closely. • Encourage oral intake if possible and assess need for intervention (e.g. dietary modifications, supplements). • If intake is persistently inadequate, consider escalating for intervention.	• Refer to Dietitian or Nutritional Support Team (NST). • Collaborate with Dietitian/NST to improve nutritional status and **manage refeeding risks**. *Do not refer when no benefit is expected (e.g. imminent death).*

Table 1.15 Simple Management Plan for Managing Malnutrition

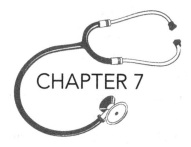

CHAPTER 7

NURSING SKILLS AND KNOWLEDGE

This is an essential part of your journey to become a competent nurse. Trained nurses are very well versed in these skills—so much so that part of your competency also depends on how well you are able to perform these skills. The *faster* you master these skills, the *more confidence* you will have in nursing your patients.

INSERTION OF NASOGASTRIC TUBE (NGT), NGT FEEDING, AND GASTRIC DECOMPRESSION

Before you are instructed to insert or use an NGT, understand the indications for it. An NGT is a tube that is inserted from the nostril to reach the stomach. It is thus an external tube that has access to the stomach and its contents. An NGT is primarily used for two reasons.

1. Tube/enteral feeding
2. Gastric decompression

I will not be teaching you the step-by-step procedure that your nursing school would probably have taught you. Instead, I will put up an algorithm that is *adapted* from the MOH clinical practice guidelines on the next page for you to ensure that the NGT is in place and ready for use.

Please note that it is *not* always necessary for a chest X-ray to be done to confirm placement. Also, please note that you can continue to use the tube for *feeding* if the pH of **gastric** *contents* (green, bilious looking) is between 5–7 when patient is on gastric pH-altering drugs. Drugs like omeprazole (a proton-pump inhibitor) can alter the acidity (increase pH) of the gastric fluid. However, do not hesitate to approach the physicians for consult or imaging when you doubt the position of the NGT and feel that it requires adjustment.

Note: In patients with gastric outlet obstruction, you may need to advance the NGT further (about 10cm) if gastric aspirates are obtained earlier than expected and minimal in quantity. Gastric decompression may not be adequate as the tube may have just passed the gastro-oesophageal junction.

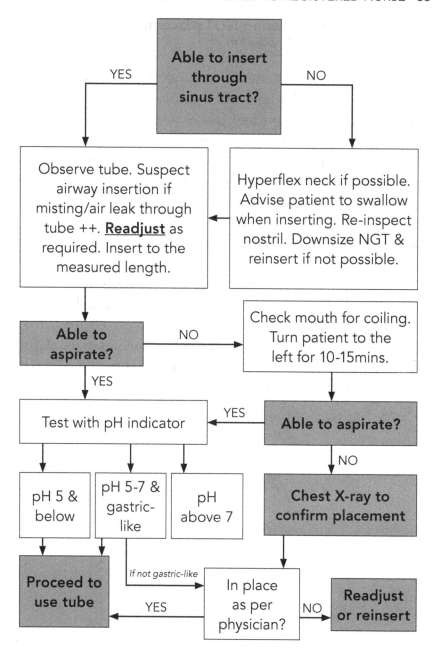

Table 1.16 NGT Insertion Algorithm[43]

---

43   Ministry of Health Singapore, *Nursing Management of Nasogastric Feeding in Adult Patients: MOH Nursing Clinical Practice Guidelines 1/2010* (Singapore: Ministry of Health Singapore, 2010), 42.

Essentials on Interpreting NGT placement
Section co-written with **Dr. Tang Si Zhao**

While interpreting X-rays is not expected of nurses, learning how to do so can benefit and improve patient care. As we understand what is an ideal placement of an NGT through a radiograph, we can then be more confident in assessing whether the NGT position compromises patient's safety. This makes complete sense as NGT insertion is one of most commonly performed procedures by nurses.

Basic Chest X-Ray (CXR) Anatomy
The salient anatomical structures to be identified on a CXR done for NGT placement are the **carina, left and right main bronchi.** You should be aware of the expected course of oesophagus (usually not visible on CXR as it is collapsed) in the midline, which courses slightly to the right, connects to the gastro-oesophagus junction, and then the stomach (sometimes can be seen as bubble, just below the left hemidiaphragm) as well.

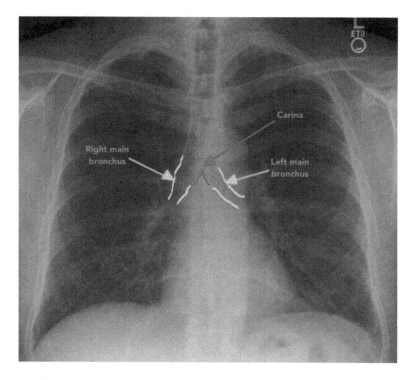

Figure 2: Basic CXR anatomy

Note: The gastric bubble is visible just below the left hemidiaphragm.

The carina is the bifurcation point of the trachea which divides into the left and right main bronchi. The correct pathway of NGT should follow the course of oesophagus and bisect the carina, as shown in the image below. The NGT appearance is like a line, due to radiopaque marker line on the tube. The tip of NGT should be advanced until it reaches the stomach, and it is recommended to place the tip at *least 10 cm* beyond the gastro-oesophageal junction (GEJ).[44]

---

44   Jain B. Pillai, Annette Vegas and Stephanie Brister, "Thoracic Complications of Nasogastric Tube: Review of Safe Practice," *Interactive Cardiovascular and Thoracic Surgery* 4, no. 5, (2005): 429–433.

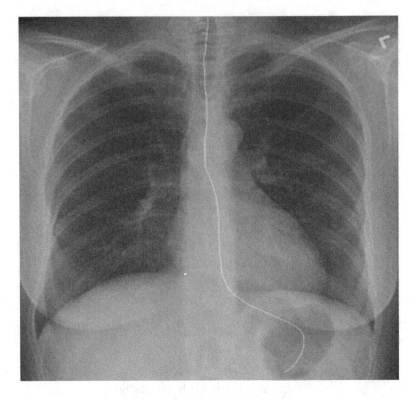

Figure 3: Satisfactory NGT position (within the stomach)

You should also ensure that the NGT tip is discernible, and it is included within the extent of CXR. In some NGT, it has a proximal side lumen/'hole'/'eye' which needs to be placed within the stomach as well. The proximal side lumen is usually visible as a short segment of NGT marker line breakage, as demonstrated in the image below. Note that this NGT has an additional radiopaque cap at its tip, which aids in tip visualisation.

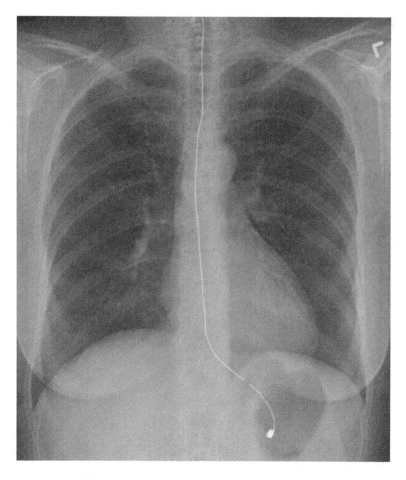

Figure 4: Satisfactory NGT position (with tip visualisation)

Note: The proximal side lumen and tip are in the stomach.

Common pitfalls in NGT insertion

1. **Accidental placement into the bronchi**. More commonly found inserted to the right main bronchus, as it provides a more direct pathway compare to left bronchus. The NGT should be withdrawn and reinserted again.

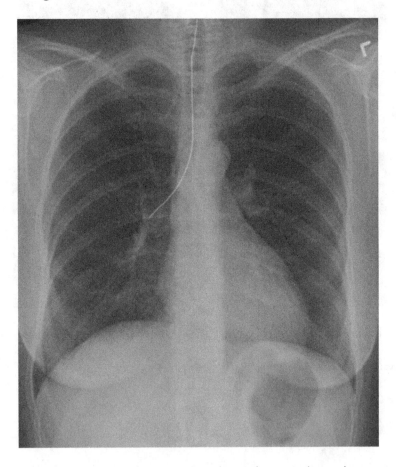

Figure 5: NGT placement in the right main bronchus

2. **Malpositioning of the tip or proximal side hole.** The tip of the NGT is placed within the oesophagus or at GEJ. This can cause reflux and induce nausea and vomiting. Further advancement of the tube is required.

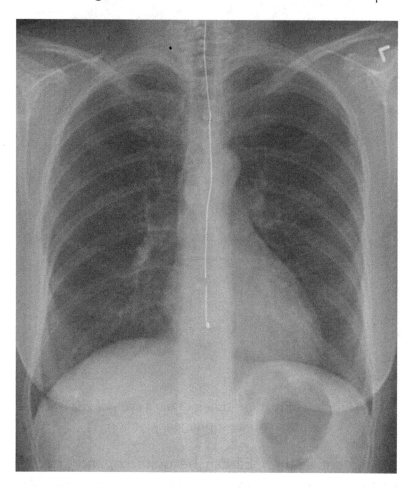

Figure 6: NGT tip in the distal oesophagus

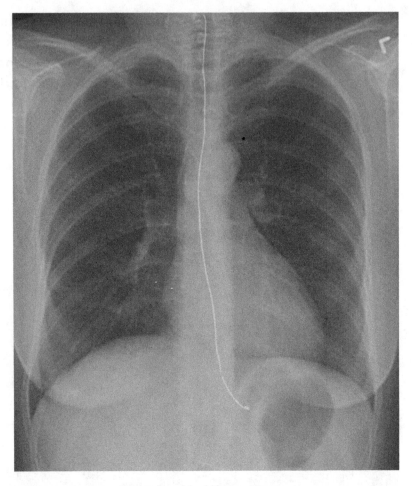

Figure 7: Proximal lumen ('hole'/'eye') of NGT
at gastro-oesophageal junction

Placement at the GEJ can be quite common in clinical practice. The NGT tip is in the stomach, but the proximal side hole is in the GEJ. Further advancement is advised for optimal placement.

3. **NGT coiling in the oropharyngeal region**. The insertion was thought to have advanced through to the oesophagus but the tube turns out to be looped. Checking the patient's mouth prior to a radiograph could have saved an unnecessary X-ray.

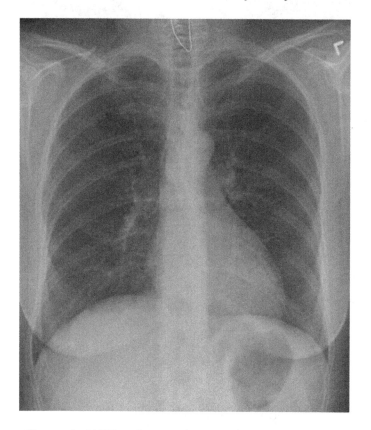

Figure 8: NGT coiling in the oropharyngeal region

Part of the NGT is visualised as a loop in the oropharyngeal area, which is suggestive of NGT coiling. Withdrawal and reinsertion should be done.

4. **Coiled configuration of the NGT at the distal part**. The tip placement is in the stomach but the NGT is coiled. There may be a need for readjustment if the tube is not patent as it is kinked.

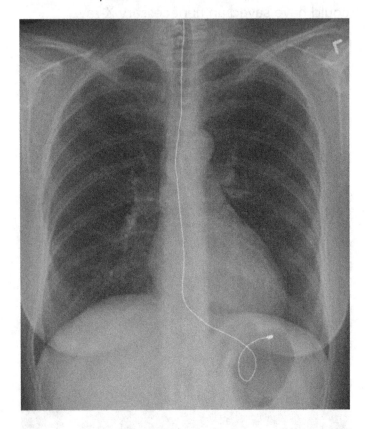

Figure 9: NGT coiled in stomach

Key features for assessing NGT placement on CXR

- The CXR coverage should include upper oesophagus down to below the diaphragm.
- The NGT should follow the expected course of oesophagus in the midline, down to the level of the diaphragm.[45]

45   Graham Llyod-Jones, "NG Tubes – Position," last accessed April 5, 2019, https:// www.radiologymasterclass.co.uk/tutorials/chest/chest_tubes/chest_xray_ng_ tube_anatomy

- The NGT should bisect the carina.
- The NGT tip, and proximal side hole (if present) should be placed below the diaphragm.
- The NGT tip should measure at least 10 cm beyond the GEJ.

If any of the listed features is absent or there is any doubt with the NGT placement, opinion from your senior or clinician should be sought.

Take note of:

- History of hiatal hernia. It is notoriously hard to insert the NGT tip into the infradiaphragmatic portion of stomach.
- History of surgeries involving the stomach (e.g. gastrectomy with oesophago-jejunal anastomosis, subtotal gastrectomy, Roux-en-Y reconstruction, etc.) The anastomotic site has a higher risk of perforation compared to normal stomach.
- Disorders involving the GEJ (e.g. achalasia).

The list above is not exhaustive and they are meant to be kept in mind. Difficulty in insertion and its associated complications are higher in patients with these background conditions. For patients with such background, discussion with a skilled clinician before commencement of NGT insertion is a prudent approach.

Assessing optimal placement of NGT on CXR is a valuable skill to have in the arsenal of your clinical practice. Be aware that in rare instances, NGT placement can lead to serious complications. Despite the aid of CXR, if there is persistent resistance encountered during NGT insertion attempts, prompt escalation to clinician for consideration of other navigating or image-guided insertion methods is highly recommended.[46]

---

[46]   Mahir Gachabayov, Kubach Kubachew and Dmitriy Neronov, "The Importance of

Feeding Tubes

There are different types and uses of feeding tubes, yet the function remains the same—to provide nutrition for the patient. The main types of enteral access include:

1. Naso-gastric tube (NGT)
2. Naso-jejunal tube (NJT)
3. Percutaneous endoscopic gastric (PEG) tube
4. Percutaneous endoscopic jejunal (PEJ) tube

As the names suggest, these tubes access the stomach or the jejunum. The type of tube chosen would depend on the condition of the patient. If the patient had part of his stomach removed (partial gastrectomy), then it would make more sense that the surgeons insert an NJT or a PEJ.

Otherwise, what we need to know about feeding tubes are the two different materials typically used for the NGT. The more commonly seen NGT would be a Ryle's tube, made from polyvinylchloride (PVC). It is only for short-term usage and more economical than a silicone NGT. The recommended duration of use of PVC is only **two weeks** because it is more rigid and tends to cause mucosal ulceration much more easily. Mucosal breakage or ulceration is the main reason why silicone NGT should be used if the patient is expected to be on long-term NGT. This is because silicone is a softer material. Silicone NGT is recommended for use up to 2-3 months or when otherwise advised as per institution's protocol.

Lastly, always ensure that the tubes are in the correct anatomy before use and always maintain its patency through diligent flushing after use.

Note: Do not confuse the recommended duration for NGT with other tubes. Non-NGT tubes are designed for long-term usage and can be even used longer than 3 months or until tube failure (e.g., blocked tube or tube dislodgement).

Chest X-Ray during Nasogastric Tube Insertion", *International Journal of Critical Illness and Injury Science* 6, no.4 (2016): 211–212.

Additional Note: It is not advisable to flush or administer feeds/medications through jejunal tube via gravity alone. Jejunal tubes are longer and narrower, and frequently cause blockages if not flushed via the bolus method (pushing the plunger of the feeding syringe).

WOUND CARE

Having a good knowledge of wound management is essential to becoming a competent nurse. Very often, only the basic principles of wound care and aseptic technique are being taught in school. However, managing wounds go beyond just placing a dressing over an injury. We also need to have a basic knowledge of the different types of wound products and learn how to use them appropriately for different types of wounds.

Principles of Wound Management

The general aims of acute or traumatic wound management[47] are:

- Facilitate haemostasis
- Exudate control
- Control microbial burden/growth and removal of debris

Where bleeding is concerned, we should stop the bleeding first before applying any dressing on the wound so as to effectively prepare the wound bed for healing. However, if bleeding is profuse, consider using a pressure/elastic adhesive bandage or manual compression (using fingers to apply pressure to the bleeding point) to achieve haemostasis.

Additional Note: In some cases, it may require calcium alginate dressings, silver nitrate cauterisation, or suturing to arrest the bleeding.

---

[47] Keryln Carville, *Wound Care Manual* (Western Australia: Silver Chain Foundation, 2017), 78.

Wound healing is optimal when the wound bed is *moist*—not too wet or too dry. This is the basis of exudate control. A very drying environment encourages scabbing, which slows tissue regeneration, even though it acts as a barrier against external contaminants. Scarring can result due to this impaired healing process. On the other hand, an overtly wet environment causes maceration of the surrounding tissues and delays wound healing. Wet environments also tend to encourage bacterial growth and skin breakdown. Always aim to achieve a *balance of moisture* when deciding on your wound products.

Usage of antimicrobial and antibiotics treatment can also help with managing the microbiological burden that hinders healthy tissue growth. Waste or dead products can become foreign bodies to the healing wound and obstruct healthy tissue growth.

Learning how to manage wounds effectively requires an on-going process of learning and applying evidence-based practices. What is taught here would probably allow you to handle simple superficial wounds with ease. **All nurses** should be able to handle wounds like abrasions, skin tears, and simple incisional/laparoscopic wounds. However, wounds that are complicated, extensive, and non-healing, (e.g. arterial or venous ulcers, wound dehiscence, wounds with deep tissue/organ involvement) would require consults to your wound specialists depending on the aetiology and state of the wound as there may be extensive repair that needs to be done before the wound can heal.

✓ **Clinical Tips**
On wound cleansing and dressing procedure

- Offer analgesia prior to wound cleansing as needed. Superficial wounds tend to be extremely painful due to involvement of nerve endings.
- Wet dressings as needed to aid in atraumatic removal of old dressings. This is essential in preserving growing, young, and delicate tissue involved in wound recovery.
- Inspect and assess wound to decide on treatment plan or next course of action before procedure.
- Ensure sufficient cleansing agent and dressing materials before commencing procedure.
- Maintain sterility by adhering to "clean-to-dirty" or "inside-to-outside" principle as much as possible.

Basic Wound Assessment

While we do our best to maintain and create conditions that are optimal for wound healing, each wound responds to the treatment differently. Part of the nursing role includes monitoring for progress (presence of granulation and epithelisation) or deterioration of the wound (e.g. redness, swelling, purulent discharges, etc). Evaluating the condition of the wound is crucial for determining the effectiveness of its current treatment, or the need for a new management plan. The nursing role on the ground is to flag up these issues *early*, should interventions appear to be ineffective.

To be able to perform a basic assessment of wounds, there are a few terminologies that require your understanding.[48,49]

---

[48]   Karen Zulkowski, "Wound Terms and Definition," *WCET Journal* 35, no. 1 (2015): 22–27.
[49]   Joseph E. Grey, Stuart Enoch and Keith G. Harding, "Wound Assessment," *The BMJ* 332, no. 7536 (2006): 285–288.

- **Epithelialising Tissue.** Pinkish tissue that typically advances from the wound edge. It is the new skin that will cover and protect the wound.
- **Granulation.** Bumpy, red, "beefy" connective tissue seen on the wound bed. Bleeds easily as it is vascularised. It is the tissue which epithelial cells migrate on to form new epithelial tissue.
- **Slough.** Non-viable tissue that has a yellow to brown appearance.
- **Necrotic Tissue/Eschar.** Dead and devitalised tissue that needs to be debrided off for wound healing to take place. Eschar is described as dry, black, and hard necrotic tissue.
- **Maceration.** Peri-wound tissue that is overly-hydrated, giving a white appearance. Macerated skin is fragile and can breakdown easily. It delays wound healing.
- **Undermining.** Destruction of the tissue underneath the wound margin. The wound cavity is larger than what is seen on the surface.
- **Purulent Exudates.** Yellowish discharges from the wound that may be foul-smelling. It is made up of inflammatory cells and tissue debris.

Basic Wound Management

To help you understand what to look out for in wound healing, I will briefly lay out a popular framework that is used to guide wound clinicians in chronic wound management (wounds that do not heal in an orderly and anticipated time frame). This will hopefully aid you in your learning process as you integrate your knowledge on wound healing.

TIME Framework[50]		
Tissue	**Assessment** Non-viable or necrotic tissue, foreign bodies, suspected biofilm or slough	**Management** Various methods of debridement to remove non-viable tissue: **Surgical/sharp**: Scalpel **Chemical**: Antimicrobials **Autolytic**: Hydrocolloids/ occlusive dressings **Mechanical**: Scraping
Infection/ **I**nflammation	**Assessment** • Aetiology of the wound (infective and non-infective causes of inflammation) • Clinical signs of infection (e.g. surrounding redness, hyper-granulation, purulence)	**Management** Systemic antibiotics Topical antimicrobials (e.g. dressings with antimicrobial effect)
Moisture Imbalance	**Assessment** The presence of wound exudates (evidence of maceration on wound edges versus dehydrated wound bed)	**Management** • Moisture absorption if there is too much exudates (e.g. highly absorptive dressings, NPWT) • Hydration of tissue (e.g. hydrogels, exudate locking dressings)

50   Rhiannon L. Harries, David C. Bosanquet and Keith G. Harding, "TIME for an Update," International Wound Journal 13, supp. S3 (2016): 8–14.

Epithelial Edge Advancement	**Assessment** • Reduction of wound area • Wound contraction	**Management** • Promote healthy wound edge (i.e. not macerated, not dry) • Treatment modalities like skin grafting (usually done by Plastic Surgery), debridement, NPWT, and hyperbaric oxygen therapy

Table 1.17 TIME management for wounds

Types of Wound Care Product Categories

The next section will list the types of wound care products and describe their materials and functions.[51, 52, 53, 54, 55, 56, 57] Only those highlighted **bold** in the table below will be described in greater detail as other dressing types may be beyond what is expected of a student/transiting nurse. However, do research on those not highlighted, as it will definitely benefit you when you start work.

---

[51]   Smith & Nephew, "Advance Wound Management," accessed 27 November 2018, http://www.smith-nephew.com/key-products/advanced-wound-management/.

[52]   Systagenix, "Our Products," access 27 November 2018, http://www.systagenix.co.uk/our-products.

[53]   Coloplast, "Wound Care Products," accessed 27 November 2018, https://www.coloplast.com.au/products/wound-care/.

[54]   Mölnlycke, "Wound Management," accessed 27 November 2018, https://www.molnlycke.sg/products-solutions/wound-management/.

[55]   Mölnlycke, "Mepilex Dressings," accessed 27 November 2018, https://www.molnlycke.sg/products-solutions/mepilex-dressings/.

[56]   3M, "Tegaderm," accessed 27 November 2018, https://www.3m.com/3M/en_US/company-us/all-3m-products/~/All-3M-Products/Health-Care/Medical/Tegaderm/?N=5002385+8707795+8707798+8711017+8711738+3294857497&rt=r3.

[57]   Urgomedical, "Products," accessed 27 November 2018, http://www.urgo.co.uk/4-products.

Primary Dressings	Secondary Dressings
• Gauze • Tulle Gras (TG) • Antimicrobials—silver (Ag), iodine and other antimicrobial impregnated dressings • Polyurethane foam • Hydrocolloid • Hydrogel • Calcium alginate • Gelling fibre/Hydrofibre • Others—creams & ointments	• Dry dressings • Moisture-vapour permeable adhesive film dressing • Elastic bandage • Triangular bandage

Table 1.18 Primary and Secondary Dressing Categories

In this section, some of the wound products that are commonly encountered in the clinical area are briefly discussed.

*Disclaimer: Please note that products listed here are **not exhaustive** and they are mentioned for the purpose of broadening your generic product knowledge. These comprise the more commonly seen products in Singapore's public healthcare institutions and many other good products may be left out. What is mentioned here **does not favour any brands over another**. Observations and opinions may become obsolete as products change and/or new evidences arise. Please exercise good clinical judgement and utilise these dressings carefully.*

Primary Dressings
(Sterile) Gauze
Types/Variations: Gauze/Gamgee/Ribbon Gauze

Gauze

- Woven fabric, typically made of cotton or a combination of absorbent materials. It is available in various brands.
- Used for cleansing and dressing of the wound.
- Can be used as a protection over minor wounds or as a *secondary dressing* for absorbing highly exudative wounds.

- **Gamgee** is an alternative for wounds with larger areas and/or high exudates.
- **Ribbon gauze** can also be used as a packing for surgical/cavity wounds when soaked with a antimicrobial.

Tulle Gras (TG)
Examples: JELONET◊/BACTIGRAS◊/UrgoTul/UrgoTul AG

JELONET◊

- Paraffin open weave gauze dressing that is manufactured by Smith & Nephew.
- Dressing tends to stick to wound surface if only a single layer is used or if there is insufficient paraffin on the tulle gras.
- Suitable for shallow wounds, typically abrasions and minor cuts with low to medium exudates. If used on its own, it does not absorb significant amounts of exudates.
- **BACTIGRAS◊** is essentially JELONET◊ but with bacteriostatic and bactericidal effect (impregnated with chlorhexidine acetate). BACTIGRAS◊ can be suitable if there is a suspicion of bacterial infection (for treatment and prophylaxis), but bear in mind that the level of antimicrobial contained is quite small.

UrgoTul

- Combination dressing—petroleum jelly and hydrocolloid (also known as lipido-colliod dressing) impregnated polyester mesh manufactured by Urgo Medical.
- Dressing can be removed easily with little trauma to the wound.

- Suitable for shallow wounds—typically abrasions and minor cuts with low to medium exudates.
- **UrgoTul AG** is essentially UrgoTul but with bacteriostatic and bactericidal effect (silver-containing). UrgoTul AG is suitable when there is a suspicion of bacterial infection (as treatment or prophylaxis).

Antimicrobials

Examples:
INADINE™/IODOFLEX◊ Pads/IODOSORB◊ (Paste/Gel/Ointment/Powder)/Other silver, iodine, and antimicrobial containing dressings

INADINE™

- INADINE™ is a low-adherent fabric with polyethylene glycol base that contains 10% povidone-iodine impregnated into a synthetic fabric dressing manufactured by Systagenix/KCI™.
- Dressing removes easily due to its base.
- Suitable for shallow wounds, typically in ulcers, due to the tendency for ulcers to become infected due to poor vascularity.
- Can be considered for desloughing wounds via chemical debridement.
- Also suitable for drying of wet gangrene, especially in DM foot.

IODOFLEX◊/IODOSORB◊

- **IODOFLEX◊ Pads** is similar to INADINE™ but is produced by Smith & Nephew. It contains cadexomer iodine, which acts through a *sustained release* of iodine as opposed to povidone iodine. Cadexomer iodine is ideal for desloughing of necrotic tissue.
- **IODOSORB◊ Paste/Gel/Ointment** is often used in wounds with unequal shapes and sizing which are

difficult to dress with woven fabric. It works better on dry wound beds as they contain some moisture.

- **IODOSORB◊ Powder** is often used in uneven or extensive areas of wounds (e.g. multiple moisture-associated denudation) that are difficult to keep dry and in place by typical primary dressings. It is activated when in contact with moisture/exudate.

Polyurethane Foam
Examples: *Mepilex®/Biatain®/ ALLEVYN◊ Non-Adhesive Foams*

- **Mepilex® Non-Adhesive Foam** is a polyurethane foam dressing with a layer of silicone adhesive designed for medium to high exudative wounds. It is produced by Mölnlycke®.
- Contact layer with silicone adhesion for ease of removal without damaging skin.
- Suitable for burns as well as pressure ulcers.
- Can be used as a secondary dressing.
- Due to its property of redistributing pressure, it is also used to offset pressure from areas of bony prominence or high pressure.
- Mepilex also comes in **Mepilex® AG**, with antimicrobial effects. It also comes in various shapes and modifications. For instance, **Mepilex® Border Sacrum** which has a water-proof silicone border to provide a strong seal around the sacrum, and **Mepilex® XT**, which has higher exudate capacity compared to its predecessor.
- Also available from brands like Coloplast (**Biatain® series**) and Smith & Nephew (**ALLEVYN◊ series**). These brands also have foam dressings with silicone borders, water-proof properties, or anatomically friendly shapes.
- When using foams, pressure redistribution properties are ideal, especially when used for pressure ulcers or

over areas of bony prominence. Not all foams available have that property. Use alternatives wisely.

Hydrocolloid
Examples: DuoDERM® (Extra Thin/CGF)/ Comfeel® Plus Transparent/ Stomahesive®/ Brava® (Powder/Paste)

- **DuoDERM® Extra Thin** is non-breathable adhesive hydrocolloid dressing. It is waterproof and produced by ConvaTec. **Comfeel® Plus Transparent** is a hydrocolloid dressing produced by Coloplast.
- Suitable for desloughing via means of autolytic debridement (softening of necrotic tissue and liquefaction of slough by moisturisation).
- **DuoDERM® CGF** has a cushion layer that provides mechanical and thermal protection. The foam layer also allows additional exudate management. Duoderm CGF is, however, not water-proof.
- **Stomahesive® and Brava® powder/paste** are different forms of the hydrocolloid dressing and are usually used for ostomies. The Stomahesive® series is produced by ConvaTec whereas the Brava® series is produced by Coloplast.

Secondary Dressings
Dry Dressings
Examples: PRIMAPORE◊/ Mepore®

- **PRIMAPORE◊** is a low-adherent pad with soft breathable cover manufactured by Smith & Nephew.
- Suitable as a secondary dressing or as a primary dressing for shallow wounds like abrasions with low to medium exudates.
- Also available as **Mepore®** from Mölnlycke.
- Applying a gauze with breathable medical adhesives taped around like a window works in a similar way as well.

Moisture-Vapour Permeable Adhesive Film Dressing

Examples: *Tegaderm™ Transparent Film/Tegaderm™ Film Dressing with Pad/OPSITE◊ Post-Op/ OPSITE◊ Film/ OPSITE◊ FLEXIGRID◊/ OPSITE◊ Spray*

- **Tegaderm™ Transparent Film** is a thin water-resistant adhesive film. Tegaderm™ is manufactured under 3M™. It is breathable, transparent, and provides a barrier to external contaminants.
- **OPSITE◊ Film** serves a similar function. The OPSITE◊ series is produced by Smith & Nephew. **OPSITE◊ FLEXIGRID◊ Film** allows the film to be cut into the shape and size that is required.
- **Tegaderm™ Film Dressing with Pad** has an added soft dressing on the transparent film. The pad serves to absorb a small amount of exudates. **OPSITE◊ Post-Op** serves a similar function but with a thicker non-adhesive pad to manage exudates.
- **OPSITE◊ Spray** is a spray that produces a transparent and quick-drying film. As it is not easily removed, it is more suitable for dry/minimally exudative wounds (sutured wounds, minor cuts and abrasions). It can also be used on unbroken blisters.

Elastic Bandage

- Elastic cotton bandage, more commonly known as crepe bandage, provides light compression and tissue support. It also secures the primary or inner dressings.

Triangular Bandage

- Multi-purpose non-elastic bandage that can be folded and manipulated for different shapes and sizes.
- Typically used to secure limbs and joints to immobilise fractured sites. Can be used as a temporary arm-sling.

Antibiotic Creams/Antibiotic Ointments
Examples: *Mupirocin/Tetracycline (Cream/Ointment)*

- Judicious use of antibiotic cream or ointment is advised due to its hydrating properties and growing antibiotic resistance.
- When used in wound beds, it is important to assess if the wound bed is wet or dry. Remember, the optimal condition for wound healing is a moist environment.
- Creams are water-based preparations whereas ointments are oil-based preparations. The difference is the duration it stays on the skin. Oil-based preparations last longer as it is harder to be removed (by perspiration, friction, etc).
- Generally, ointments should be avoided for hairy areas due to its risk of developing folliculitis.
- Tetracycline ointment is one of the commonly used antimicrobial ointment in our public healthcare institutions. Typically, **tetracycline 3%** ointment is used for all parts of the body except the face and more sensitive areas. **Tetracycline 1% ointment** will be used for facial skin and sensitive areas.

In order to help you understand the various *categories* of wound products better, I have come up with a simple summary table on the next page. They are sequenced according to their ability to control exudates. Please take note that this list is, again, **not** entirely exhaustive.

TYPE OF DRESSING	EXUDATE CONTROL	FEATURES	ANTIMICROBIAL FORM?
Hydrogel	None	Hydrates very dry wounds and can provide auto-lytic debridement and desloughing.	Yes E.g. SilvaSorb® Gel
Creams & Ointment	None	Provide moisture with antiseptic properties to dry wounds.	Yes E.g. Tetracycline ointment
Film Dressing	None	Protection with water-proofing. Can act as a reinforcement layer. Good for isolating wounds.	None
Tulle Gras/ Lipidocolloid	None–Low	Contact layer, which provides a moist healing environment. Atraumatic removal of dressing.	Yes Silver-based: UrgoTul AG. Iodine-based: INADINE™.
Hydrocolloid	Low–Moderate	Occlusive dressing, good for isolating wounds. It is used for desloughing (autolytic debridement). Can also be used for protecting the peri-wound.	None
Gauze	Moderate–High	Manages simple exudative wounds. Used for cleansing.	None, unless soaked with an antimicrobial like iodine solution or chlorhexidine.
Foam	Moderate–High	Pulls out exudate and provides gentle cushioning. Good for pressure ulcer prevention.	Yes E.g. Mepilex® AG
Calcium Alginate/ Gelling fibre	Moderate–High	Manages highly exudative wounds. Alginates have haemostatic effect, but gelling fibres do not.	Yes Calcium alginate: ALGISITE◊ AG. Gelling fibre: AQUACEL® AG.

Table 1.19 Summary Table for Wound Product Categories

With the understanding of the overarching principle of wound care, basics of wound assessment, as well as familiarisation with different categories of wound products, the RN can better monitor the progress or deterioration of the wounds and work collaboratively with the various specialists to achieve a better care for the patients.

STOMA CARE

Stoma actually just means "opening" in the Greek language. In nursing, the commonly used term "stoma" is more accurately an *enterostomy*—which means an opening of the digestive tract. The most commonly encountered enterostomies are the colostomy and ileostomy. Colostomy involves part of the *large intestines* opening onto to the abdominal wall and hence you can expect the waste matter to be more faecal-like. As for ileostomy, it would involve the *small intestines* instead which is more proximal in the digestive system and hence the waste would be more fluid and bile-like. Nurses should be able to monitor for stoma health, peri-stoma skin status, as well as the output from the enterostomy. A healthy stoma should look *pinkish* and not blackish or gangrenous. Peri-stoma skin should not look red and irritated by the waste materials (also known as "contact irritant dermatitis"). Enterostomal discharges should not look bloody or tarry (small amount of blood is acceptable in the early post-op period after creation of stoma). Referral should be made as soon as possible to a stoma nurse for any suspected stoma or peri-stoma complication.

A stoma or enterostomal nurse should be on board for every newly-created stoma to ensure that comprehensive caregiver training (CGT) and counselling is done for the patient and his/her caregivers. Nurses on the ground should be familiar with the different stoma drainage application systems and measuring/estimating the correct sizing for the drainage system. Should leakages happen outside office hours, nurses on the ground need to be competent to handle them.

Here are some of the terminologies and products[58] that you need to be familiar with to be comfortable taking care of stomas.

- **Stoma application system—one-piece versus two-piece.** In one-piece systems, the base plate (or wafer) is attached to the stoma bag. In two-piece systems, the stoma bag is detachable from the base plate.
- **Base plates—flat versus convex.** Convex base plates have a protrusion. This is used for stoma openings that are "sunken" below or in line with the level of peristomal skin.
- **Base plates—mouldable versus non-mouldable.** Mouldable base plates do not need to be cut to size. Their inner edge can be moulded, or rolled, to fit. Otherwise, *all* other base plates need to be cut to fit.
- **Stoma size.** Base plates come in different sizes and they have a range that you are allowed to cut/mould to maintain adhesion. 45mm is one of the most common sizes in our local context.
- **Barrier/stoma (hydrocolloid) paste.** Multi-purpose paste used to even out skin creases to prevent leakages.
- **Stoma (hydrocolloid) powder.** Used to manage denuded skin.

Understanding the usage of different products is good knowledge when you start nursing ostomates with varying stoma sizes and appearances.

---

[58]   Janice C. Colwell, "Selection of pouching system," in *Ostomy Management*, eds. Jane E. Carmel and Janice C. Colwell (Philadelphia: Wolters Kluwer, 2016): 120–130.

MONITORING OF INVASIVE LINES, TUBES, AND DRAINS

In general, if your patient has a line, drain, tube, catheter, or anything on him that is not natural, think in terms of how the device is being placed and how it serves the patient. As they are foreign bodies, we need to watch for the possibility of infection developing around it or entering the body through it.

In that same line of thought, think about what you should see and what you should not (e.g. is a red streak along an IV cannula normal, or could it be phlebitis?). Also, if the object has already served its purpose, can it be taken out as soon as possible to prevent infection?

Indwelling Urethral Catheter (IDC)

An IDC is a tube that drains the urinary bladder. It has an inflatable balloon for the IDC to remain seated inside the bladder to prevent accidental dislodgement. Its purpose is to drain out urine and could be used for the following reasons:

- Monitoring of urinary output for critically ill patients, or patients who need close monitoring of fluid status
- Management of acute or chronic urinary retention
- Continuous bladder washout for patients with gross haematuria, or in the early post-op period after some Urological procedures
- Urinary diversion to allow perineal wound healing

Similarly, like the feeding tubes, it is important to know the materials[59,60] of an IDC to understand their function and

---

59   UroToday, "Designs—Intermittent Catheters," accessed 30 November 2018, https://www.urotoday.com/urinary-catheters-home/intermittent-catheters/description/designs-intermittent-catheters.html.

60   UroToday, "Designs—Indwelling Catheters," accessed 30 November 2018, https://www.urotoday.com/urinary-catheters-home/indwelling-catheters/description/designs.html.

recommended duration of use. This goes hand-in-hand with monitoring for possible complications that arise from the use of an IDC.

- **PVC/nelaton.** Only suitable for intermittent catheterisation, and not appropriate to leave in the urinary tract. It does not have an inflatable balloon and is too hard and rigid for prolonged use. Ideal for manual bladder washout.
- **Latex/silicone-coated.** Recommended for short-term catheterisation of up to *one month*. Infections and irritations to the urothelial mucosa tissue tend to be more prevalent with latex use. Encrustations also tend to develop on latex as well. An advantage of latex as compared to silicone is its cheaper price. However, most short-term IDC now are silicone-coated, as pure latex has become an unpopular choice due to its frequent complications. It is good to note that with silicone-coated latex catheters, the life-span is not extended as the thin layer of silicone is susceptible to wear and tear.
- **Hydrogel-coated/100% Silicone.** The preferred material for patients who need long-term catheterisation, as these can be changed up to once every *three months*. Patients who repeatedly fail "trial off catheter" (TOC) and have opted for long-term IDC use are suitable for this. It is also the recommended material for suprapubic catheterisation (SPC). Hydrogel becomes smoother when rehydrated, hence, it can reduce friction in the bladder or urethra. This makes it a preferred choice of material when the catheter is to be kept in the urinary tract longer.

As an IDC is a foreign object, always monitor for signs and symptoms of a urinary tract infection. An infection of the urinary tract can precipitate cloudy and foul-smelling urine together with other signs and symptoms of infection (fever, tachycardia, and raised white-cell count). Also monitor for haematuria as a possible sign of urothelial tissue damage.

Note: Care of patients with urinary catheters is important to prevent urosepsis, especially for the immunocompromised, elderly, and immobile patient. Urosepsis is often associated with high mortality rates.[61]

Intravenous (IV) Access

IV *insertion* is a skill that you are not allowed to practice as a student nurse. However, you will realise very early in your RN career that setting IV cannulas and administering IV medications are often part and parcel of your daily work! As a student nurse, you are allowed to manage and care for IV access. Hence it is important for you to be able to identify the complications of IV access and IV therapy.[62]

Phlebitis

It is the inflammation of a vein. Localised redness and pain are often the first signs. Please inform your staff nurse to re-site the IV cannula if the pain becomes persistent or when swelling and a streak formation occur. Apply ice to the site and apply anti-inflammatory cream to ease the pain and swelling. Do take reference from a visual infusion phlebitis score to assess the severity of phlebitis.

Infiltration

It is the leakage of IV fluids into the surrounding tissue instead of being infused into the veins. High osmolality of IV fluids, movement or dislodgement of IV cannula, and presence of phlebitis can cause infiltration. Please inform your staff nurse to re-site when it is evident that the fluid is not flowing into

---

[61]   Om Prakash Kalra and Alpana Raizada, "Approach to a Patient with Urosepsis," *Journal of Global Infectious Disease* 1, no. 1 (2009): 57–63.

[62]   Lisa Bonsall, "Complications of Peripheral I.V. Therapy," last modified 9 February, 2015, https://www.nursingcenter.com/ncblog/february-2015-(1)/complications-of-peripheral-i-v-therapy.

the vein (i.e. no back-flow when aspirating with a syringe, and swelling of surrounding tissue when normal saline is flushed into the cannula).

Extravasation

It is the infiltration of a *vesicant* to the surrounding tissues. A vesicant can cause severe irritation to the surrounding tissues, leading to necrosis. It may present as pain at the infusion site, swelling, and in serious cases there may even be blistering. Common vesicants include IV potassium chloride, high-concentration dextrose solutions, and dopamine. If it happens, stop the infusion immediately but keep the IV cannula for a possible administration with an appropriate antidote of the vesicant after informing the physician. Elevate the limb while awaiting physician review.

Central Lines

These are also known as central venous catheters (CVCs) which are placed into a large vein. The tip lies either in the superior vena cava, or the inferior vena cava. They can be very useful for various reasons. Being positioned in a large vein, medications and parenteral nutrition that are otherwise caustic (or with high osmolality) to the peripheral veins can be administered more safely through the central lines. These lines can remain in place for a longer duration than other IV access devices, which is useful for patients needing chemotherapy. Further, these lines can also be used for drawing blood as well as monitoring of haemodynamic status (e.g. central venous pressure) for critically ill patients.

A peripherally inserted central catheter (PICC) is typically inserted via the basilic vein or the cephalic vein in the arm. The central venous catheter (CVC) is usually inserted either from the internal jugular vein or the subclavian vein in the neck; or the femoral vein in the groin.

When handling central lines, one needs to be stringent to prevent the risk of developing a line infection and serious sepsis. Measures include adhering strictly to an aseptic technique to administer infusion therapy, especially in administering total parenteral nutrition (TPN), and a weekly antiseptic cleansing and dressing change of the puncture site to prevent infection. Should a line infection be suspected, the line has to be removed and a tip culture (tip of the central line will be cut off and sent to lab) would be taken, together with blood cultures.

Drains

Drains are typically used to remove unwanted body fluids/waste or collections within a body cavity. The cavity could be from an intra-abdominal space or it could be from a wound cavity caused by debridement/incisions. However, in the case of chest tube drainage for pneumothorax, it would be used to drain out *air* from the pleural cavity, preventing the lungs from collapse and respiratory failure.

Also, you need to know the difference between an **active** and a **passive** drain. An active drain uses a vacuum bottle to suction out the bodily fluids. A passive drain has no vacuum and uses only gravity to drain out the bodily fluids. This means that passive drains should always be placed below the drainage site, to allow gravity to work. It is also important to detect when the vacuum of an active drain is gone, as it will now function as a passive drain. There is usually an indicator for suction and the loss of suction may indicate a need to change the drainage bottle.

As nurses, we will need to highlight to the physician if there are abnormally high or low amounts of drainage or discharges which relate to clinical signs and symptoms. For instance, if 300ml of bloody discharge from a surgical drain were to occur within an hour, and the patient presents with sudden hypotension or tachycardia and shortness of breath, there would be a high suspicion for overt bleeding and fluid resuscitation along with other interventions would probably be needed. These clinical manifestations were discussed in the previous chapter, *"Nursing Monitoring and Management"*.

Note: Ensure lines, tubes and drains are secured well as accidental dislodgement can happen. Take good care of the peri-tube skin through regular inspection, cleansing, and dressing as it could be a site of infection.

CARE OF PALLIATIVE PATIENTS
Section co-written with **Katherine Lim Ci Hui**

Some journeys do not always end up in recovery. At a certain point in healthcare, there will be a need to call for palliation and focus at the end-of-life.

Communication is important when taking care of palliative patients. Details such as their character, outlook on life, values, cultural and religious beliefs, family background, social life, and coping enable us to know more about the patient and their family members, their goals of care and wishes. This ensures that the *care will be congruent* and effectively communicated to all family members. Any issues or queries such as unrealistic expectations can be addressed so that goals of care can be aligned, and patients' wishes are respected. It is important that this discussion is done sooner, rather than later, when patient still has the mental capacity to make decisions. Family members and loved ones can be prepared for the patient's possible deterioration and death and any bereavement risk can be identified.

Advance Care Planning

Advance Care Planning (ACP) is an important platform for effective communicative to take place.

ACP is the process of planning for patients' future health and personal care. It allows patients to have a conversation with their loved ones to share their personal values and beliefs, how they will affect healthcare preferences in difficult medical situations. It also allows patients to nominate a healthcare spokesperson to follow their wishes and make decision on their behalf in the event when they can no longer speak for themselves.

Advance Care Planning is **not legally binding** and the care preferences can be **changed anytime**. It is good to initiate discussion about goals of care whenever the patient's condition changes/deteriorates. Furthermore, anyone can be trained to be an ACP facilitator and initiate the discussion, including nurses.[63]

End-of-life Care

Below are the common symptoms experienced by patients at the end of life:

- Pain
- Dyspnoea
- Delirium & agitation
- Constipation
- Nausea/vomiting
- Secretions
- Fever

Pain

Pain is a common symptom experienced by patients nearing the end of life. It can affect patients in all aspects of their lives. It is important to recognise and assess patients' pain, which includes not only the physical symptoms but also the social, psychological and spiritual distress which arise from the pain itself.

---

[63] Living Matters Advance Care Planning, "About ACP," accessed 10 May, 2019, https://www.livingmatters.sg/advance-care-planning/about-acp/.

Pain Assessment

Apart from utilising the pain scales that we have discussed in the subchapter, *"Pain"* in *"Nursing Monitoring and Management"*, we can obtain a comprehensive pain history by using the acronym, **SOCRATES**. **SOCRATES** is used to evaluate the nature of pain that a patient is experiencing.

- **S**ite

  - Where is the location of the pain? Is it localised (concentrated in a specific area) or diffused (spread out)?

- **O**nset (pattern and mode of onset)

  - Did the pain occur rapidly, gradually or instantaneously?
  - Is the pain present continuously or intermittently?
  - Is the pain getting worse or better? When did the pain become worse or better?

- **C**haracter

  - Ask the patient to describe the characteristics of the pain (e.g. stabbing, dull, sharp, cramp-like, burning, aching, pulling, or squeezing type of pain)

- **R**adiation

  - Determine if the pain radiates (spreads to a specific location or direction).

- **A**lleviating factors

  - Does anything make the pain better?
  - Has analgesia been used to control the pain?

- <u>T</u>iming

  - When did the pain first begin?
  - How long did it take for the pain to be relieved?

- <u>E</u>xacerbating Factors

  - Does anything make the pain worse?

- <u>S</u>everity

  - Pain is subjective. The best way to assess severity is to ask patients to rate themselves and ask if the pain interferes with normal activities or sleep.

Types of Pain

There are different types of pain a patient can experience. Knowing the characteristics of pain is essential as this will determine the types of analgesia and management to be given to patient.

- **Nociceptive pain**

  - Pain related to damage of somatic or visceral tissue due to trauma or inflammation
  - Characteristics: Aching, dull, squeezing, cramping
  - Examples: Gout, osteoarthritis

- **Neuropathic pain**

  - Pain related to damage of peripheral or central nerves
  - Characteristics: Sharp, needle-poking, stabbing, burning
  - Example: post-herpetic (post-shingles) neuralgia

Breakthrough Pain

Breakthrough pain consists of transitory exacerbations pain which can occur despite being on a baseline opioid regime (e.g. fentanyl patch and morphine sulphate tablet).

- A sudden increase in pain which occurs in patients who already have chronic pain from their underlying conditions.
- Usually lasts for a short time.
- The characteristics and location could be the same as the usual pain.
- Can occur with stress, illness and activities, such as exercising or coughing.

When breakthrough pain occurs, an additional dose of opioid may be prescribed and given to reduce the suffering of the patient.

Dyspnoea

Dyspnoea can be caused by different mechanisms such as pneumonia, aspiration, anaemia, and pleural effusions. It is commonly seen in patients with cancer and end stage pulmonary/cardiac disease.

Patients who experienced dyspnoea are often found to have anxiety at the same time which further exacerbates their sensation of breathlessness. Both breathlessness and anxiety are linked very closely to each other. Therefore, this results in patients going into a cycle of increasing breathlessness and anxiety.

To assess the nature and severity of dyspnoea, **SOCRATES** assessment *can be used as well*. Common pharmacological management of breathlessness at end-of-life includes opioids such as morphine and fentanyl.

As for non-pharmacological managements of breathlessness, they include:

- Aiming a cool fan towards patient
- Sit up the patient
- Pursed lip breathing

Common Misconceptions Regarding Use of Morphine

When starting morphine or other opioids, there might be resistance from patient and their family members due to its negative association with addiction and end-of-life. Tackling these queries is important to help them see the benefits of using morphine.

- **Addiction.** Patient and their family members might be concerned that morphine can cause addiction. It is important to explain to them that as the patient has ongoing pain or dyspnoea, morphine is being used as a medication for symptom relief which will not result in addiction. In contrast, for healthy individuals who do not experience any symptoms, the likelihood of addiction after taking morphine would be high.
- **Effectiveness.** There are worries that morphine will not work eventually when the patient's pain/dyspnoea worsens. There is actually no ceiling for the dosage of morphine. The dosage of morphine can be increased accordingly as their symptoms worsen.
- **Use of morphine = end-of-life.** Morphine is *not* just for people who are dying. It is commenced when a patient's pain cannot be adequately controlled with mild to moderate analgesia such as Paracetamol or Tramadol. It is indicated for symptom relief.

Delirium and Agitation

There are various causes of delirium and agitation in palliative patients. Some of the reasons include:

- Brain metastasis
- Constipation
- Electrolytes imbalance such as hypercalcaemia
- Pain
- Infection
- Urinary retention

Causes for delirium should be identified and treated accordingly. Identification of the causes can guide appropriate treatment:

Management of delirium and agitation can include:

- Managing electrolytes imbalance
- Treating infection with antibiotics
- Ensuring regular bowel clearance and offering regular toileting
- Assessing pain and targeting it with pain relief medications
- Ensuring adequate fluid intake
- Frequent re-orientation to time, place, person.
- Ensuring glasses or hearing aids are in place for patients who require
- Placing familiar objects near patient
- Minimising noise and sleep interruption at night to promote sleep hygiene

Constipation

In palliative patients, constipation is one of the symptoms that they are prone to develop. Use of opioids, decrease in mobility, reduction in fluid intake, tumour obstruction, and hypercalcaemia are all contributing factors to constipation among them.

Symptoms to look out for include:

- Abdominal bloating, discomfort, or distension

- Early satiety or decrease in appetite
- Reduction in bowel output
- Change in bowel patterns
- Spurious diarrhea—passing watery stools frequently
- Dilated rectum during rectum examination

Ensuring regular bowel clearance is essential as it not only affects comfort, but it can cause a myriad of problems such as a loss of appetite and even intestinal obstruction. Treatment of constipation typically involves the use of laxatives which is discussed in the subchapter, *"Need to Know Basic Pharmacology"*.

If constipation still occurs despite the patient being on regular oral laxatives, medications can be inserted through rectum for a faster or more effective relief.

Care in the Final Hours

Knowing what to expect in the final days or hours can help people to get ready for the death of their loved ones and hence giving them comfort and allaying them of their anxiety. As nurses, we should communicate with family members regarding changes which may happen to their loved ones in the final hours. We should also find out whether they have any important cultural/religious beliefs and customs which are important at the end of life (e.g. no touching of the body for several hours after death).

Signs to look out for nearing the end of life

- **Reduction of oral intake.** Family can offer ice chips or swab the mouth and lips to keep them moist. Risk of choking should be explained to family members should they want to feed to patient. Some might request for IV drip after seeing their loved ones' oral intake reduced or unable to swallow, however, this may not be beneficial for patients at the end of life.

The use of IV drip at the end-of-life may cause:

- Fluid overload, resulting in generalized swelling of the body due to multi-organ failure.
- Buildup of respiratory tract secretions and breathlessness due to ineffective airway clearance.

  - **Increasing drowsiness**. Patients may spend more time sleeping, become less alert and more withdrawn. They may become more confused, sometimes agitated, restless, or start having some hallucinations. However, patients can still hear and feel even if they are no longer able to speak or speak coherently. Hence, as nurses, we should encourage family members to continue to touch and talk to the patients even if they no longer respond.
  - **Decreased urine & bowel output**. Urine can become more concentrated in colour.
  - **Changes in breathing pattern**. They may start gasping for air, present with shallow breathing, and observed to have Cheyne-stoke breathing (a pattern of breathing that is characterised with progressively rapid breathing that results in a temporary stop and the cycle repeats).
  - **Changes in extremities**. Patients' hands and feet may turn cold, blue, or mottled in appearance.
  - **Death rattle**. Occurs when saliva or other fluids start to accumulate in the throat and upper airways. Management can include positioning patients laterally, oropharyngeal suctioning and the use of subcutaneous hyoscine butylbromide infusion/injection.

At a point in our nursing career, we are bound to take care of patients at the end-of-life even if it is not in a hospice setting. As nurses, we need to be effective communicators and sensitive to the different needs of these patients and other patients around them.

NEED-TO-KNOW BASIC PHARMACOLOGY

To be able to function as a nurse taking cases, you *need* to be able to recognise the drugs that you are giving to your patients. On top of that, you would need to *at least* know what the drugs are used for and the effects they produce (i.e. drug class). However, there are so many different drugs being used each day that as a student/transiting nurse, you may not know where and how to begin.

Note: https://www.mediview.sg is a useful website and resource for nurses to identify the physical appearance of medications. It contains images of most medications kept in government hospitals and is updated as the formulary changes. It may be especially beneficial for nurses who work in the community, reviewing medications that are kept in pill boxes.

To help you kickstart your learning, I will list down the common drug classes and medications you are likely to encounter. You should read up on them and see how these drugs are being prescribed to the patients that you encounter during your clinical placements. While learning, be mindful of medications:

- that should **not** be crushed (e.g. enteric-coated/modified-release medications)
- that should be served pre-meal, with meal, or after meal (e.g. omeprazole and aspirin)
- that should be served in a time-sensitive manner (e.g. vancomycin, gentamycin) if drug levels need to be monitored

You will be able to get the hang of medication administration as you become familiar with these drugs. With a basic drug familiarity, you will find it easier to learn and understand drugs that have more complicated mechanisms.

Note: Serving medications is also more than just adhering to the "5 rights". By understanding the "right reason" for the medication, we can help to prevent errors that may cause harm to the patient. For instance, should we blindly serve a regular dose of antihypertensive to a patient with deteriorating blood pressure? We must understand that the wellbeing of patients is dependent on nurses.

Generic Drug Class	Common Examples
Analgesic	Paracetamol, Tramadol, Diclofenac, Etoricoxib, Naproxen, Pethidine, Fentanyl, Oxycodone
Antipyretic	Paracetamol, Ibuprofen
Antibiotic	Augmentin, Ceftriaxone, Metronidazole, Piptazo (Piperacillin/Tazobactam), Clarithromycin, Ciprofloxacin, Vancomycin, Meropenem
Antiemetic	Metoclopramide, Ondansetron
Antihypertensive	• Calcium Channel Blockers (-dipine) [*Amlodipine*] • Beta-Blockers (-lol) [*Bisoprolol*] • Angiotensin II receptor antagonist (-sartan) [*Lorsatan Potassium, Telmisartan*] • ACE inhibitors (-pril) [*Enalapril Maleate*]
Diuretic	• Thiazides (*Hydrochlorothiazide*) • Loop diuretics (*Furosemide*)
Anti-cholesterol	• Statins (*Simvastatin*) • Fibrates (*Fenofibrate*)
Hypoglycaemic Agent	• Insulin (rapid, regular, intermediate, and long-acting) • Sulfonylureas (*Glipizide*) • Biguanides (*Metformin*) • Gliptins (*Sitagliptin, Linagliptin*)
Antiplatelet	Aspirin, Clopidogrel, Ticagrelor
Anticoagulant	Heparin, Enoxaparin, Warfarin, Rivaroxaban
Gastro-protective Agent	Omeprazole, Famotidine, Magnesium Trisilicate
Laxative	Lactulose, Sennosides, Bisacodyl, Fleet Enema, Polyethylene Glycol (PEG)

Electrolyte Replacement	Sodium Chloride, Potassium Chloride, Magnesium Sulphate, Calcium Gluconate
Supplement	Vitamin B12, Vitamin B complex, Ferrous Fumarate/Gluconate/Sulphate, Vitamin D, Folic Acid
Corticosteroid	Prednisolone, Hydrocortisone, Budesonide
Sympathomimetic	Adrenaline, Dopamine, Phenylephrine
Benzodiazepine	Lorazepam, Diazepam

Table 1.20 Common Drugs

TRANSITION-TO-PRACTICE

Transition-to-Practice (TTP) is a time when you are expected to exhibit what you have learnt in all the years of your nursing school and show that you are able to provide competent and quality nursing care. However, the most important thing is that once you graduate, you will shoulder the responsibility of taking care of your patients. It is therefore, essential that you take an active role in seeking as many learning opportunities as possible to ensure your smooth transition to become an RN.

Do take time to revise the previous sections on "Clinical Years" as it contains valuable foundational nursing knowledge.

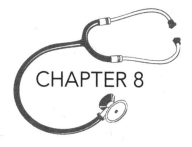

CHAPTER 8

YOUR PRECEPTOR

As you begin to take up responsibilities as a staff nurse in-charge for your patients, a preceptor will be there to guide you. He or she will teach you to become a good staff nurse. This time round, however, you will no longer be accompanied by your fellow nursing school mates, instead you will be working alone with your preceptor and other nursing staff that you are assigned to.

Understanding how to work with your preceptor or whoever that is guiding you will be **key** to performing well during your TTP.

Understand that precepting is an additional task that your preceptor has

This means that they have their daily assignments to fulfil **while** guiding you. As a student nurse, you will need to be prepared to be the one initiating learning outcomes with your preceptor. Not all assigned staff may be experienced in teaching or guiding. They might also be swamped by their own assignments and responsibilities. Your learning may be limited as a result of all these.

Furthermore, your allocated preceptor may not always be around due to their annual leaves, sick leaves, maternity/

paternity leaves, family-care leaves and training leaves. If you know that your main preceptor will not be around in the ward for a large portion of your TTP, you need to highlight to your hospital facilitator as well as the ward sister *as soon as possible*. This will minimise the chance of you finding yourself without proper guidance.

In short, your learning and ability to adapt to the ward *depends on you*. Do not feel like you are limited by your circumstances, but know that you can make things happen if you discuss them with the appropriate people.

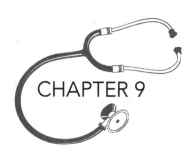

CHAPTER 9

CRUCIAL LEARNING OUTCOMES

Very often, you will be asked by your clinical instructors or preceptors: "What do you want to learn or achieve for this posting?" Many a time, students do not know how to answer this question, as they are completely new to the setting and do not quite know what to expect. Riding on this struggle, here are *four* important pointers to help you plan out your learning outcomes.

1. Learning hospital protocols

Learn about hospital-wide protocols that you will need on a day-to-day basis, such as receiving new admissions, ordering of diet, insertion of NGT and verification of placement, IV medication administration (including blood product administration), giving subcutaneous and intramuscular injections, transferring patients to ICU, discharging patients, and last office procedures. These protocols are usually standardised across the whole hospital regardless of ward and discipline, and you will encounter them in your daily work as a staff nurse in charge.

2. Learning ward practices

After learning the hospital protocols, it is good to learn about your individual ward practices. They may have different practices in nursing care, for example, some wards may practise sponging patients at 6 a.m. (meaning that this is done by night shift staff instead of the morning shift). Such differences will affect the way you plan for your nursing care.

As a student nurse, you are expected to follow and comply with the ward practices. The faster you can adapt, the deeper you can go in your learning.

3. Learning the management of common acute diseases

In every discipline, there are usually diseases that are more common to that discipline. For example, when being attached to an Acute Medical Ward, you may frequently encounter cellulitis, pneumonia, or patients being admitted for giddiness. If you are attached to an Orthopaedic Ward, you will see patients with fractures, including many hip fractures, who will be on weight-bearing restrictions and require various mobility aids. In an Acute Surgical Ward, you will encounter patients with various presentations of abdominal pain, or abscesses of the trunk, and will find yourself accompanying patients to and back from scans or the Operating Theatre. When you aim to understand the management of *common* acute problems early on during your posting, you allow yourself more space and confidence to learn about cases that are less common and more complex. TTP is already a stressful event—by reducing stress through early preparation, you have more room for development during your attachment.

4. Master nursing routines of your ward

To become proficient at what you are doing, you need to pick up the routines of the ward as soon as possible. By the end of week 1, aim to be very familiar with the routines of junior work (role of enrolled nurse) and in-charge (IC) work (role of RN). Be able to answer the question: What duties or tasks will the EN and RN start off their shift with? Which tasks are less urgent and can be done later? Without this understanding, you will not be able to anticipate the nursing routines required, or prioritise the more urgent and important needs. In this phase of TTP, preceptors and managers are not looking at how much textbook knowledge and theory you know. They are looking for nurses who have **both** the clinical knowledge and ability to work. Having theoretical knowledge without the ability to work on the ground is useless in a clinical setting.

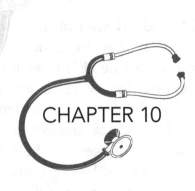

CHAPTER 10

NURSING & MEDICAL HIERARCHY

Another important background preparation to start off as an RN is to understand how the hierarchy of nursing and medicine work. Doctors and nurses are often required to work closely together. By having a clearer picture of the chain of command, it will help you to navigate through the seemingly complex maze of hospital operations.

NURSING HIERARCHY & PROGRESSION TRACK
Enrolled Nurse (EN)

Enrolled nurses are nurses who perform their duties under the supervision of an RN. One main differentiating role between the RN and EN would be the restriction on medication administration. ENs typically take on a more supportive role for the RN, but may assume more responsibilities under institutional protocols and career development. ENs have a different career track that does not overlap with the RN. They are, however, often encouraged to further their studies and transit to a RN.

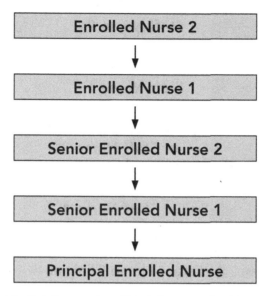

Table 2.1 Promotion Track for Enrolled Nurses

Note: A Patient Care Assistant (PCA) is **not** a nurse. Their role is to mainly help the RNs and ENs with simple tasks, so do not expect them to perform at the same level as an EN.

Registered Nurse

For a staff nurse to go up to a level of a senior staff nurse and beyond, he or she is expected to be able to manage more complex issues like manpower, service quality, clinical audit, and quality improvement, beyond discharging their duties in caring for their assigned patients. They may be given additional roles to lead. To go on further to the different specialised tracks would require the senior nurses to fulfil the different components of their tracks (e.g. nurses interested in the educator track would want to involve themselves with the clinical instructor role, planning in-services, and developing teaching plans for student and new nurses).

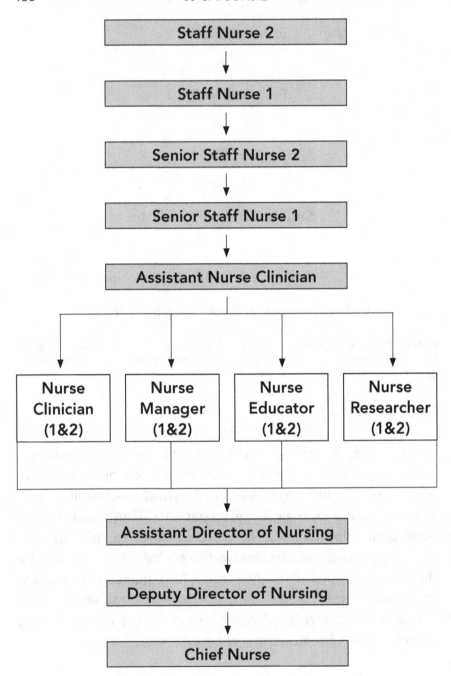

Table 2.2 Promotion Track for Registered Nurses

Note: Your Reporting Officers are the ones that give you your performance rating. They are at managerial level and above–i.e. Assistant Nurse Clinician level and above.

Additional Note: Advance Practice Nurse is more of a role than a rank. They are in the clinical track and perform at the nurse clinician level. Specialty care are experienced nurses and can start from the senior staff nurse level.

MEDICAL HIERARCHY & PROGRESSION TRACK
Section co-written with **Dr. Ryan Tan Choon Kiat and Dr. Rebecca Goh Wenhui**

House Officer (HO)

Known as the Do-it-all, these newly minted graduates from various universities are the members of the medical team that you will see most often on the wards. A large part of their duties centre on clerking new admissions, ordering up "changes" (medications, investigations, diet orders, referrals to other disciplines), and preparing the patient for discharge. They are often the ones performing simple procedures on the wards such as IDC insertion and blood-taking, and preparing the discharge documents. As their duties are largely confined to the wards, they are expected to know their inpatients' medical conditions at their fingertips and update their seniors promptly of any changes. They are usually the first-line doctors to attend to any sudden deterioration in their patients' conditions, initiate basic orders to stabilise the patients before further and more definitive decisions are made by the seniors.

Medical Officer (MO)

The Sandwich class. After completing a year of Housemanship and being deemed worthy of progressing up the ranks, the promoted Medical Officer heaves only a quick sigh of relief upon realising a different set of responsibilities awaits. Compared to HOs, the MOs' responsibilities have greater variance depending on the specialty they are posted to. For instance, a MO in Surgery is expected to be the first doctor to arrive in the Operating Theatre to receive the first patient of the day, and hence may not complete the ward round with the rest of his team. It should be noted that in certain specialties, such as Neurosurgery, Medical Oncology, or Intensive Care Medicine, the MO may be the most junior ranking member in the team as these specialties do not take in HOs as part of their team.

Apart from looking after patients in the wards, MOs may also see patients in the outpatient clinics under the supervision of their Registrar or Consultants. MOs in Surgical disciplines may also assist in the Operating Theatre or Endoscopy centres.

For the care of inpatients, MOs are usually the second-line of contact (especially on-call) if the HO is uncontactable, or if the HO needs to escalate the situation to a senior.

You will also encounter the term Residents, who are under a specialty training programme (Residency). Residents in their first and second year of training (i.e. R1s and R2s) usually function at the level of a MO. Still, this terminology varies between departments and hospitals due to reasons such as manpower allocation, length of specialty training, etc. It will therefore be good to clarify with a senior.

Registrar, Resident Physician (RP)

The Seniors. The Registrar is in his final years of Residency training, after which he may assume the post of a Consultant.

Resident Physicians are not part of a residency programme, but are experienced, competent and skilled in their relevant specialties. After working in a certain specialty for a couple of years, some MOs may choose to carry on working in their departments as a permanent staff without going through the traditional consultant training pathway. Many RPs function as a Registrar, leading ward rounds, receiving referral letters on behalf of the team, or performing surgical procedures independently. As such, they are also highly valued members of their departments.

Consultant (Associate Con., Con., Senior Con.)

The Boss or Know-it-all. Consultants have completed specialty training, and can practise independently without supervision. All patients admitted to public healthcare institutions are assigned a Consultant who will ultimately be responsible for their care. Consultants oversee the work of the junior doctors in their team and often also teach during the morning rounds. The best time to speak to them directly would be during the morning rounds, although many questions about patient care can be saved for the end of rounds and directed to the more junior members of the team. Over time, you will notice that different Consultants have different working styles and different ways they wish to conduct rounds. For example, some Consultants will do a "paper round" with their team, where they briefly run through all patients on the team list and identify important overnight events or lab results, which can sometimes help the "physical round" of going to see patients be quicker and more efficient. Some Consultants may prefer to skip the "paper round" and instead view each patient's medical chart and lab results while at each patient's bedside.

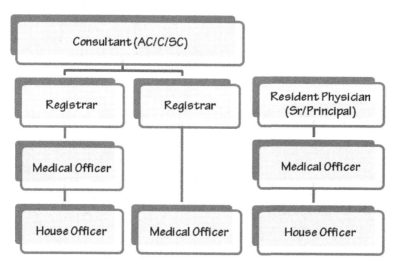

Table 2.3 Promotion Track/Team Structure for Medical Doctors

The Grand Scheme of Things

Do not belittle your role. Your hard work will play a significant part in helping the House Officers and Medical Officers, and in turn benefits the entire medical hierarchy and more importantly, the patients themselves. Healthcare may sometimes feel like a thankless job and your doctors may not always show their gratefulness and appreciation towards the many things you do, menial or glorious these tasks may be. Perhaps it may be the build-up of fatigue from long working hours, having another unstable patient to attend to, or a difficult next-of-kin to communicate with, which may have unfortunately robbed even their cheerful demeanour away, let alone their ability to compliment your efforts with a sincere "Thank you!".

Regardless, remain steadfast that your service is ultimately to your patients and every effort, whether it is noticed or appreciated, counts towards their overall well-being. Our medical colleagues who contributed to this book can strongly attest to that.

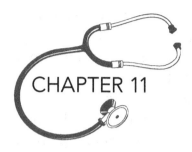

CHAPTER 11

NURSING ROUTINES

Routines vary from shift to shift. As a student nurse, you will be expected to master both A.M. and P.M. shifts. Night shifts, on the other hand, are more for exposure at a student nurse level. Different hospitals have different shift durations and shift rosters, depending on the schemes that they adopt. Flexi-hours are adopted by some institutions where the employees work shorter hours for the particular shift while some adopt the compressed work week model.[64]

MORNING SHIFT

Morning shifts usually start at 7 a.m. and can end at 4 p.m. Here are the tasks that you can expect:

- Receive handover from night shift (updates of conditions/overnight events, latest treatment plans, vital signs, I/O over 24-hours, and blood test results)
- Assisting in ADLs (showering, ambulation, diet/feeding, elimination)
- Taking vital signs, BSL, and I/O monitoring

---

[64] Ministry of Manpower Singapore and Ministry of Community Development and Sports Singapore, *Flexible Work Arrangements* (Singapore: Ministry of Manpower, 2001), 2–9.

- Serving morning medications (in particular, 8 a.m. medications, as the quantity of medication served is more than in other shifts)
- Doctors' rounds, updating medical teams about significant observations or changes in patients
- Performing procedures
- Sending patients to diagnostic investigations, haemodialysis, or Operating Theatre
- Meal break
- Documentation, communication, and follow-up of loose ends (documentation includes: updating the nursing care plan; nursing assessment including wound charting, nursing education, updating access lines; updating I/O charts, significant events during shift; and listing follow-up actions to be taken by the next shift)
- Discharging patients (Collating discharge summary, prescription, Medical Certificate, outpatient follow-up appointments ("TCUs"), and memos for the patient, if any)
- Handing over to the next shift

Taking over a comprehensive and thorough report from the night shift is important—the IC needs to know what happened the day before, the plans for the patient today, any issues that occurred overnight (along with what corrective actions were rendered) and whether the morning bloods have been taken and dispatched. If there are any important issues that were not appropriately managed, highlight and discuss them immediately. ADL and morning medications usually happen concurrently upon taking over from the night shift.

Nurses tasked with the junior role will fulfil their junior tasks throughout the shift, including taking and updating vital signs, BSL, and I/O. In the junior role, one plays a supporting role to IC. The IC is still the one accountable for whether nursing tasks have been completed. Thus, if you are the IC, it is good to communicate and check with your supporting junior whether tasks have been completed as planned.

Nurse ICs will begin serving medications while awaiting doctors' rounds. Physicians may arrive on the ward as early as 7a.m. to as late as 10.30a.m. During the doctors' round, ICs are expected to provide updates or to highlight nursing issues to the medical team so that patients can have the best treatment plans. ICs also need to make sure that the charts are updated as the vital signs, I/O, and BSL trends are crucial for the doctors to make decisions (e.g. whether to increase IV hydration if the patient is in negative balance, or to titrate DM medications).

After medications and doctors' rounds, be ready to follow up on "changes" or loose ends. You may need to accompany or arrange a porter for patients undergoing diagnostic imaging (e.g. X-Rays, CT scans, or Ultrasound scans), assist in laboratory investigations (e.g. blood tests, urine/stool/wound specimen collection), and trace the input from blue-letter reviews, and other allied health reviews (e.g. PT/OT, medical social worker (MSW), dietitian, podiatry). Sometimes, there are events that are scheduled in advance, (e.g. operation scheduled for 1000H, to keep fasted and omit all hypoglycaemic agents in the morning) and you will need to ensure that necessary preparations have been made.

AFTERNOON SHIFT

Afternoon shifts typically start at 1 p.m. and end at 10 p.m. Here are the tasks that you can expect:

- Receive handover from the morning shift (updates of conditions, vital signs, I/O, and blood test results, as well as the latest treatment plans)
- Serving afternoon medications
- Facilitating transfers and accepting transfers

- Receiving admissions from Emergency Department, clinics, and Admission Office.
- Assisting in ADLs (showering if not yet done, ambulation, diet/feeding, elimination)
- Vital signs, BSL, I/O monitoring
- Follow up on loose ends, including late discharges
- Doctors' exit rounds
- Meal break
- Serving night medications
- Communication with the patient and their family members (many relatives visit after office hours)
- Facilitate caregiver training (CGT)
- Documentation
- Handover to the night shift

Serving afternoon medications is usually not as demanding as morning round medications. After the ICs have served the medications, it is usually time for patient movements (transfers) and following up of the various "changes" that have begun since the morning. There is a second round of medication serving from 7 p.m. for the night medications, which is again, not as demanding. However, you might find that you may be approached by family members more often during the afternoon shift, as most of them come to visit their loved ones after office hours. Do use this opportunity to build good relationships with your patients and their family.

Many elective admissions also arrive to the ward in the afternoon. Elective admissions are usually admitted for a specific reason or event, such as for undergoing investigations as an inpatient, or for a scheduled procedure. These patients usually arrive on the ward via the Admissions Office, and you, the RN, may be the first healthcare worker that they meet. They may not have been seen yet by a doctor before arriving to the ward, unlike admissions from the Emergency Department. For these patients, you should look out for their latest outpatient clinic documentation, or their admission form, to understand the purpose of their admission. While elective admissions tend to be less acutely unwell than admissions from the Emergency Department, they may also be frail or have multiple medical problems, so do ensure that they are promptly clerked by the medical team.

Afternoon shift is also a good time to start preparation for the next day's tasks. For instance, we can start arranging the ambulance transfer for a Nursing Home patient due for discharge the next day, start collating discharge documents for patients planned for discharge the next day (especially if the patient has been a long stayer and multiple "TCUs" and discharge documents are anticipated), and initiate pre-operative preparations. Other routines are similar to morning shifts.

NIGHT SHIFT

Night shifts start at 9 p.m. and end around 7.30 a.m. the next day. Here are the tasks that you can expect:

- Receive handover from the afternoon shift
- Serving medications (typically only medications that require round-the-clock administration such as IV fluids or analgesia, or medications that are time-sensitive in dosing, such as antibiotics)
- Reinsertion of IV lines if they are due
- Facilitating ADLs (feeding, elimination)
- Vital signs, BSL, I/O monitoring
- Tidying the common workspace and topping up of consumables
- Close I/O charts at 2359H (24H intake/output)
- Meal break
- Receive admissions from ED

- Specimen collection, especially morning bloods that are usually drawn at 6a.m.
- Documentation
- Handing over to the morning shift

Night shift routines are usually slower and less intensive as most patients are expected to be sleeping. The patient-to-staff ratio however, doubles for the night shift so as to conserve manpower for morning and afternoon shifts. Throughout the hospital, there will be fewer medical and nursing personnel around at night. During this time, services and interventions (diagnostics, surgeries, and procedures) are prioritised for the critically ill; while routine or non-urgent investigations will be reserved for the daytime. Working the night shift requires you to be fairly independent and able to make sound decisions, as you will have fewer colleagues around.

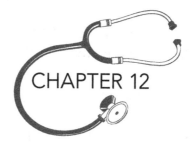

CHAPTER 12

TAKING CASES

Now, you are should be ready to start taking care of patients with your preceptor's supervision. Before you do so, let me help you with the final bits where students struggle the most because they were never really taught how to deal with them until their clinical placements.

MANAGING CHRONIC DISEASES

In Singapore, the burden of chronic diseases is set to increase due to our ageing population. These chronic diseases will accompany patients that are admitted for acute medical or surgical problems. As a RN-to-be, you should aim to learn how the different types of chronic diseases are being managed as they can interfere with the patient's recovery from their acute issues.

Here is a list of common chronic diseases that RNs should be familiar with:

- Diabetes Mellitus (DM)
- Hyperlipidaemia (HLD)
- Hypertension (HTN)

- Chronic Kidney Disease (CKD) and End-Stage Renal Failure (ESRF)
- Congestive cardiac failure (CCF)
- Cardiac Obstructive Pulmonary Disease (COPD)
- Asthma
- Hyper/hypothyroidism

Some of these chronic diseases are quite straightforward in their management, but some are not so. Thus, I will discuss **three** chronic diseases that are trickier to manage in the next sections. But before we discuss, next is a table to help you understand the management of the various chronic diseases better.

CHRONIC DISEASE	GENERAL WARD MANAGEMENT
DM	• OHGA • Insulin administration • BSL/HbA1c monitoring • DM diet
HLD	• Cholesterol-lowering drugs (usually statins) • Monitor lipid panel • Low fat diet
HTN	• Antihypertensives • BP monitoring
CKD/ESRF	• Iron supplements, phosphate binders, IV erythropoietin (commonly known as Recormon) • Regular dialysis if ESRF • Fluid restriction • Low potassium, low phosphate diet

	• Arm precautions for the arm with AVF • Monitor dry weight
CCF	• Diuretics • Fluid restriction • Low salt diet • Daily weights
COPD, Asthma	• Inhalers (reliever and preventer) • Proper inhalation technique. Assess need for space chamber • Antibiotics if infective exacerbation
Hypo/Hyperthyroidism	• Synthetic thyroid hormone/anti-thyroid medication.

Table 2.4 Summary Table for Chronic Disease Management

Diabetes Mellitus

DM is a disease of the endocrine system, and the principal organ involved would be the pancreas. DM has to do with resistance and insufficiency of insulin, a hormone released by cells in the pancreas. As such, much attention has to be paid to the monitoring of blood sugar levels (BSL). Recall in the previous section the normal and abnormal ranges of BSL and its immediate management.

Usual Orders for Blood Glucose Monitoring (BGM) & Sliding Scale:
TDS + 10PM, or Q4H

For the typical DM patient, monitoring of their BSL pre-meals and before sleeping helps in assessing if their medication regime is optimal. Q4H monitoring would be ordered when patient fasts, for example, in preparation for surgery.

Use of Sliding Scale Insulin therapy (SCSI)

The use of SCSI is something that is usually taught on-the-job. SCSI refers to a range of insulin doses to be given for a range of BSL readings. They are usually ordered in conjunction with BGM. The use of sliding scale (SCSI) is always *temporary* and, typically, Actrapid® (fast-acting insulin) is used for titration. SCSI comes in low-dose, medium-dose or high-dose, depending on the patient's size/body weight and the level of insulin requirement.

Due to changes in medical conditions, dietary restrictions for surgeries/diagnostics, or other problems that influence the BSL, SCSI will come in handy to control BSL during hospitalisation as it is easy and convenient to use to keep patient's BSL in check in the short-term.

Research has also shown that good sugar control peri-operatively produces better outcomes, such as faster wound healing and lesser post-operative complications.

Note: While using an *insulin pen*, remember to **prime at least two units** of insulin as you attach a new needle to the pen each time. In contrast, when using an insulin vial, the drawing of insulin from the vial via the syringe already primes the needle for direct injection, thus there is no need for a further priming step. The use of an insulin pen is preferred for patients with difficult in drawing out insulin from a vial (e.g. poor eyesight or lacking fine motor dexterity).

Always store your insulin pen or vial in the fridge when it is unopened to maximise shelf-life. Once used, it can be stored under normal room temperature and away from sunlight.

Managing the Diabetic Foot
Section co-written with **Acacia Neo Jia Wei**

The most frequent cause of diabetic foot ulcer (DFU) is repetitive external trauma that results in a break in the cutaneous barrier. This occurs a sequela of peripheral neuropathy and foot deformities.[65] DFU can be further complicated by infection and peripheral arterial disease (PAD).[66]

PAD can independently increase the risk of non-healing ulcers, infection, and amputation.[67] In treating DFU, nurses should learn to identify if it is a neuropathic, ischaemic, or neuroischaemic ulcer. Where infection is suspected, it is important to regularly inspect the wound and to change the dressing frequently. Wound dressings should be used in combination with appropriate wound bed preparation, systemic antibiotic therapy, pressure offloading, and diabetic control.[68]

Note: The principles of wound management were discussed in the 'Wound Care' subchapter of *Chapter 7: Nursing Skills and Knowledge*.

Dressing Application for Diabetic Foot Ulcers
Improper techniques can further compromise a foot with PAD and cause more iatrogenic wounds on the deformed foot. Below are some good pointers.

---

[65] Gayle E. Reiber, Loretta Vileikyte, Edward Boyko, Michael Anthony del Aguila, Douglas Smith, Lawrence A. Lavery and Andrew J. M. Boulton, "Casual Pathways for Incident Lower-Extremity Ulcers in Patients with Diabetes from Two Settings," *Diabetes Care* 22, no. 1 (1999): 157–162.

[66] David G. Armstrong, Andrew J. M. Boulton and Sicco A. Bus, "Diabetic Foot Ulcers and Their Recurrence," *The New England Journal of Medicine* 376, no. 24 (2015): 2367–2375.

[67] Armstrong, Boulton and Sicco, "Diabetic Foot Ulcers and Their Recurrence," 2367–2375.

[68] Paul Chadwick, Michael Edmonds, Joanne McCardle and David G. Armstrong, "Best Practice Guidelines: Wound Management in Diabetic Foot Ulcers," *Wounds International* 376, no. 24 (2013): 1–23.

- Avoid tight bandaging (pulling bandages while applying) especially around the toes as this may cause a tourniquet effect.
- Avoid creases and having overly bulky dressing.
- Avoid strong adhesive tapes on fragile skin if possible.
- Avoid using Tegaderm™ or OPSITE◊ dressing over toes and on any necrotic tissue with vascular insufficiency.

Footwear Recommendation

Patients with diabetes are encouraged to use footwear that fits, protects, and accommodates the shape of their feet. Additionally, they should be advised to always wear socks with their footwear to reduce shear and friction. Patients at high risk of ulceration (e.g. neuropathy, foot deformity) should be advised to obtain footwear advice from a podiatrist to ensure their shoes are of proper fit.

For patients with a healed plantar foot ulcer, prescribed footwear and accommodative insoles are recommended. Prescribed footwear and accommodative insoles are effective in reducing plantar pressure at the high-risk area on the foot, as these patients are vulnerable to re-ulceration.[69] Such patients are encouraged to use their footwear *at all times*, both indoors and outdoors. For patients with an active plantar diabetic foot ulcer, the podiatrist should prescribe appropriate offloading devices to heal these ulcers.

Nurses should pay special attention to the patient with a diabetic foot and seek assistance from the podiatrist especially when these patients have to start ambulating and are going to be discharged back to the community. Nurses **can save** their legs with a good judgement.

---

[69] Jaap J. van Netten, Peter A. Lazzarini, David G. Armstrong, Sicco A. Bus, Robert Fitridge, Keith Harding, Ewan Kinnear, Matthew Malone, Hylton B. Menz, Byron M. Perrin, Klass Postema, Jenny Prentice, Karl-Heinz Schott and Paul R. Wraight, "Diabetic Foot Australia Guideline on Footwear for People with Diabetes," *Journal of Foot and Ankle Research* 11, no. 2 (2018): 1–14.

Chronic Kidney Disease/End-Stage Renal Failure and Chronic Cardiac Failure

Impairment of the kidneys and heart can cause fluid retention in the body. While some of the symptoms of retention are not an emergency in themselves (e.g. uncomfortable swelling of the feet and ankles), depending on its severity and organ affected, it can lead to a life-threatening emergency (i.e. respiratory failure when too much fluid accumulates in the lungs).

Usual Orders for Fluid Restriction:
Fluid restriction (500mL, 800mL, or 1L per day)

A healthy person would require 2-3L of fluids per day. The amount of fluid restriction depends on the patient's condition (e.g. severity or presence of peripheral oedema, pulmonary congestion or cardiac function). The ejection fraction of the heart can also influence the amount of fluid to restrict.

Usually, if the patient is on dialysis, the fluid restriction is stringent as these patients can only pass little or no urine to get rid of extra water, and diuretics will have no effect on them if they are in fluid overload. Be vigilant when you hydrate patients in ESRF. One bag of 500ml of saline may be *all* the fluids the patient is allowed in a day.

Note: Fluid restriction applies to *all kinds* of fluid entering into our body, per enterally (e.g. food and liquids) or parenterally (e.g. IV antibiotics, IV fluids). Food like porridge and fruits which contain more liquid should also be cautiously taken into consideration.

Additional note: Interestingly, some long-term dialysis patients have developed a habit of drinking and eating what they love or taking extra drinks just before dialysis to make the experience of having ERSF and dialysis more manageable, since at all other times they have to adhere to restrictions.

Usual Orders:
Daily weights, dry weight (post-dialysis weight)

It is essential to accurately measure and trend the weight of the patient with fluid retention, especially the ones with

ESRF, to estimate how effective is the diuretic therapy and/or dialysis session.

Pre-dialysis weight is typically taken just prior to the dialysis or estimated from daily weights on non-dialysis days. Post-dialysis weight, sometimes also known as *dry weight*, is taken right after the dialysis session. The baseline dry weight is the ideal weight that the patient should have after dialysis when he/she is well and has not missed any dialysis sessions.

Usual Orders for patients on haemodialysis:
HD 1,3,5 or HD 2,4,6

ESRF patients on haemodialysis typically have a regime of dialysing either on Monday, Wednesday, Friday (1,3,5) or Tuesday, Thursday, Saturday (2,4,6). Many of them adapt well to such a regime and some may even continue to work in between their dialysis sessions. Sometimes, when the ultrafiltration (UF) achieved (the volume of fluid removed), is not ideal or insufficient, they may be required to dialyse again the next consecutive day.

Note: Suitable patients may opt for continuous ambulatory peritoneal dialysis (CAPD), to minimise disruption to daily activities. Patients on CAPD dialyse daily, but this can be done by themselves or by their caregivers in the community.

Diuretics
The most commonly prescribed diuretic would be furosemide. In some patients who do not respond to high doses of furosemide (diuretic resistance), you may see other diuretics such as metalozone/bumetanide being added on. One thing to note is that after you administer this medication, the patient may have a lot of urine to pass. Watch out in particular for patients that are of high fall-risk, and anticipate their need for supervision and assistance to the toilet.

It is also important to take note of the patient's blood pressure before administering diuretics, as the drawing out of fluids in a patient with low BP can worsen the hypotension. If patient's baseline BP is borderline low (SBP 90s or low 100s), discuss with the physician whether to withhold the diuretic or serve a lower dose.

Note: Not all ESRF patients are anuric.

Phosphate Binders, Erythropoietin, and Iron Supplements

As the renal function declines, the kidney's ability to regulate minerals also worsens. Phosphate, being one of the minerals that will no longer be excreted properly, is retained and can lead to high levels of phosphate in the blood. This is why you will often see *calcium acetate* ordered for these patients because it is a calcium-containing phosphate binder. However, if the patient's calcium level is also high, there may be a need to switch to non-calcium containing phosphate binder such as *lanthanum or sevelamer.*

During haemodialysis, it is expected to have some blood loss, mainly from circulation in the tubing of the machinery. Also, their kidneys are impaired and do not produce as much erythropoietin, which is a necessary hormone to produce haemoglobin. Erythropoietin, in synthetic form, is commonly known as *Recormon.* It is often administered during dialysis to help with haemoglobin production. Similarly, PO/IV iron supplements may be ordered for replacement as iron deficiency is common in renal patients. Iron supplements can also help to improve the patient's response to erythropoietin therapy.

Note: Recormon injection can increase the BP of patients, especially in ESRF patients undergoing dialysis.[70] Care has to be taken when administering Recormon to the patient. With uncontrolled blood pressure, omission should be considered to prevent the precipitation of hypertensive crisis.

---

[70] Hamid Noshad, "Blood pressure increase after erythropoietin injection in hemodialysis and predialysis patients," *Iranian Journal of Kidney Diseases* 21, no. 3 (2013): 220–225.

Arm Precaution

It is also important to note that arm precautions should be put up for the arm with AVF to avoid damaging it. BP and blood-taking should be avoided on the arm with AVF.

Chronic Obstructive Pulmonary Disease

Understand that COPD is a condition that is usually acquired by smokers and results in chronic obstructed airflow to the lungs. Their bodies adapt to the chronically reduced level of oxygen in their tissues. Thus, patients with COPD are at risk of having their hypoxic drive suppressed when given *high concentrations* of oxygen. It is good to be mindful when administering oxygen therapy to this group of patients. What is also good to note is that clinicians usually target their oxygen saturation to be at *88% to 92%*, instead of the usual 94-98% for the average person.

✓ <u>Clinical Tips</u>
On oxygen titration

- Have you read *Chapter 3: Nursing Monitoring and Management—Respiratory Rate and Oxygen Saturation?* The chapter also teaches on how to titrate oxygen therapy for COPD patients.

Inhalers

Like asthma, people with COPD may require *preventers* (i.e. LAMA [long-acting muscarinic agents] inhalers like Tiotropium) to prevent exacerbations. They may be prescribed with PRN *relievers* (i.e. short-acting bronchodilation inhalers like salbutamol) as well. These commonly seen medications, which will be described in the next section, should usually be restarted ASAP upon admission by the physician if not contraindicated.

Nebulisers

Typically, when we administer nebulisers to a patient, it is done via a nebulisation mask *with* **at least** 5L O2/min. However, for the COPD patient with COPD who **does not need** supplemental oxygen, an air compressor should be used instead, to avoid the risk of him developing hypercapnia.

Patient's Old Medications

You might have seen the phrase "restart old meds" many times and thought to yourself—what are old medications? No, it is not expired medications. It is the long-term medications that patients are already on before they come into the hospital. Sometimes, physicians may make the decision to withhold all old medications or they may restart some but deliberately omit a few medications.

Note: Do not mix up the terms—"patient's *old* medications" with "patient's *own* medication". Patient's own medications refers to the medications that they physically brought with them to the hospital. Sometimes, patients may wish to take their own supply of medications while in hospital because they have a large stock of them at home and do not wish to waste them. In some circumstances, patients may have special or rare medications (such as chemotherapy medications or immunological medications) that may not be part of the hospital's standard supplies, and hence they have to consume their own medications until the hospital pharmacy obtains a supply for them. The medications brought in by the patients or their family members can be sent to the pharmacy for medication reconciliation.

Additional Note: Be careful when you identify controlled drugs (e.g. PO oxycodone, fentanyl patch) in a patient's possession. Storage and transport of such medications can have legal liabilities, hence it is pertinent to know and abide by your hospital's protocol in managing such medications.

INTERPRETING COMMON LAB RESULTS

As a student nurse taking care of patients, it is also essential that you are able to pick out abnormal lab results that need the doctor's attention. This is also because nursing actions are usually required promptly thereafter.

Blood Glucose

As discussed in the chapter, *Nursing Monitoring and Management,* normal blood glucose level ranges from 4.0–7.8mmol/L. Blood glucose levels of *less than 4.0mmol/L* are known as hypoglycaemia. Immediate recognition with corresponding rectifying action is required. While hospitals may differ slightly in managing hypoglycaemia, a glucose-containing drink (usually dextrose powder dissolved with water) for conscious patients is almost universal. This is followed by IV dextrose administration if BSL levels still do not normalise. Close monitoring of the BSL will be required at this stage (every 15mins until normal BSL).

Note: NEVER attempt to resolve hypoglycaemia with *slower-acting sugars* like lactose (milo, milk) if dextrose powder is not available. The time required to resolve hypoglycaemia is much longer and the patient may proceed to fall into unconsciousness. You can always get fast-acting sugars like fructose from juices readily available in the ward.

Sometimes, you may encounter a *"Hi"* reading on your glucometer. This means that the BSL is out of the range of the meter's upper limit. This may signify potentially dangerous conditions of diabetic ketoacidosis or hyperosmolar hyperglycaemic non-ketotic syndrome. "Hi" readings warrant an urgent call to the physician. Prompt treatment with IV fluids and IV insulin would be required.

Haemoglobin (Hb)

Usually indicated in Full Blood-Count (FBC)

Hb measures the amount of the haemoglobin molecule in a volume of blood. Normally, it ranges from 13.1 to 17.2 grams per decilitre (g/dL) for men and 11.2 to 15.6 g/dL for women. As an RN, you need to have a rough idea how much of a Hb drop would warrant an action to be taken by the physician. The threshold for "low Hb" can sometimes be quite wide. Hb of *less than 8.0* would typically warrant a blood transfusion, especially if there is an evidence of ongoing or recent blood loss.[71] Otherwise, it would be dependent on whether the patient is symptomatic (e.g. SOB, chest pain, giddiness) or whether there is massive bleeding and recent trauma. Interpreting this result allows you to pre-empt transfusions as well as to alert the team. The RN is liable for informing the medical team if you have been notified of a critical result by the lab staff.

A rise in haematocrit value (ratio of the volume of red blood-cells to the total volume of blood) should be expected after a unit of packed-cell is given, typically about 3% and Hb should rise about 1g/dL. However, sometimes, the Hb and the clinical presentation of the patient may not tally after a blood transfusion. This may be due to a *dilution of blood specimen* (specimen taken on the arm running an IV drip) and can be recognised if there is a sudden decrease of all the cell counts in FBC from baseline, with no evidence or suspicion of blood loss. You can highlight your suspicions to your preceptor or the physicians, to avoid panic and unnecessary further transfusions without first rechecking the Hb level.

Additional Note: When transfusing blood for a patient, besides watching for possible signs and symptoms of blood transfusion reaction, also be mindful of the patient's hydration status. In many ESRF/CCF/end-of-life patients, fluid overload is often a commonly overlooked issue as physicians may get too fixated on correcting the deranged Hb. You should raise such concerns to your physicians before initiating a blood transfusion.

Potassium (K+) and Other Electrolytes

Usually indicated in Renal Panel (RP) and Bone Metabolism Panel (BMP)

Electrolytes are very important as they are essential for normal cardiac function and nerve conduction. Gross derangements should be corrected as soon as possible so

---

[71] Jeffrey L. Carson and Steven Kleinman, "Indications and Hemoglobin Thresholds for Red Blood Cell Transfusion in the Adult," in *UpToDate*, ed. Ted W. Post (Walham: Massachusetts, 2018).

as to prevent a potentially fatal cardiac event. As a nurse being notified of electrolyte changes, you should be able to understand the magnitude of the lab value and the necessary corrective actions to be taken.

If electrolytes are *lacking*, the management is relatively straightforward, as we just need to replace the necessary electrolytes. If there is a significant deficiency, then this is done intravenously. If the derangement is mild, we can consider oral replacement or consider using a hydrating drip containing the particular electrolyte. Do note in certain deficiencies such as low potassium and low sodium, it may be dangerous for the patient if their levels are corrected too quickly. Confirm with your doctor about the fluid of choice, and the rate of infusion, if you are in doubt.

However, in the case of *elevated* electrolytes, the management may not be so simple. In this section, I would like to briefly highlight how you can expect to manage a patient with hyperkalaemia.[72] This can happen quite frequently in patients with impaired renal function and is not uncommon at the ward level.

For hyperkalaemia levels of *K+ >6mmol/L*, you will be required to:

- Take a set of vitals
- Perform an ECG
- Check BSL
- Standby IV dextrose 50% and Actrapid® insulin for the physician to administer (most hospitals pack these in a "hyperkalaemia kit")
- PO or rectal Resonium may also be served
- Recheck K+ and BSL (ensure patient does not turn hypoglycaemic)

---

[72] David B. Mount, "Treatment and Prevention of Hyperkalemia in Adults," in *UpToDate*, ed. Ted W. Post (Walham: Massachusetts, 2018).

The purpose of administering IV dextrose and insulin is to shift the extracellular K+ into intracellular space, thus rapidly decreasing serum K+. This action can usually be done twice before considering means of dialysis if other treatment for possible causes of hyperkalaemia fails.

If there are new ECG changes such as tall-tented T waves, there will be a need to administer IV calcium gluconate. Calcium stabilises the cardiac membrane, opposing the effects of cardiac membrane excitability from hyperkalaemia. When there are ECG changes present with hyperkalaemia, the patient may require telemetry or closer monitoring because of the increased risk of cardiac arrest.

Note: *There are some institutions that allow nurses to administer 100ml of IV dextrose 20% with insulin via the volumetric pump, without waiting for the physician to arrive. Do check your hospital's hyperkalaemia protocol before carrying out your orders.*

If *K+ <6mmol/L*, but elevated, you may be required to administer sodium polystyrene sulfonate (or known as Resonium, available in per oral or as per rectal forms), to remove K+ by means of the gut.

Severe electrolyte imbalances can be potentially life-threatening if not treated fast, hence it is important that as a student nurse and soon to be RN, you must know what is happening and how to handle such conditions.

Note: *Always check if sample is haemolysed or not. Haemolysed samples would give spuriously elevated K results.*[73]

---

[73] Calgary Laboratory Services, "Effects of Hemolysis on Clinical Specimens," accessed 29 November 2018, http://www.calgarylabservices.com/lab-services-guide/specimen-collection/hemolysis.aspx.

MANAGING NON-MEDICAL ISSUES
Section co-written with **Chew Tee Kit**

In every healthcare setting, healthcare providers need to acknowledge and understand that health and well-being is *closely associated* with many other non-medical problems like social, financial, and psychosocial issues.

In the clinical setting, it is not uncommon to quickly brand any form of social or financial concerns to the medical social worker (MSW) and abdicate ownership of such problems. As a result, nurses and doctors do not always have a very clear idea dealing with non-medical issues. Without a certain level of competency to manage these non-medical problems, we will fail to fulfil our duties to promote health.

> ## Case Example 1
>
> *Mr. Tan was a 76-year-old man who came into the hospital after he developed fever for 3 days with lethargy. Blood profiles and chest X-ray revealed community-acquired pneumonia. His response to IV antibiotics was good and infection was resolving on day 2 of hospitalisation. The medical team intended to discharge him on the next day with PO antibiotics.*

This is a very typical case that would be admitted to hospital under the acute internal medicine discipline. The expectation is: *patient comes in with a problem, receives treatment, and goes home.* Furthermore, with frequent hospital bed crunches and hospital administrators pushing for "discharge before noon", medical and nursing teams would be more than happy to activate "D-1" in preparation for patient to transit back home.

Now, let us complicate the above scenario.

Case Example 2

Mr. Tan was a 76-year-old man who came into the hospital after he developed fever for 3 days with lethargy. Blood profiles and chest x-ray revealed community-acquired pneumonia. His response to the initial IV antibiotics was poor and antibiotics was escalated. His infection settled down on day 5 and the medical team intended to discharge him after completion of 7 days of IV antibiotics. However, the nursing team highlighted mobility and ADL difficulties as Mr. Tan could not walk steadily or wear clothes without assistance, and he **would be at home alone for most of the day**. PT/OT was engaged to review patient but the patient could only tolerate sitting out of bed. The patient's family was very concerned as Mr. Tan **used to be fully independent**. Inpatient rehabilitation was recommended and the family agreed with the plans as they had sufficient MediSave coverage.

The second case example illustrates the journey of many patients, especially the elderly, who come into the hospital. New issues surface, or it is discovered that the patient had not actually been coping well at home. A post-acute plan for recovery is offered with hopes of returning them back to pre-morbid levels. This case assumes that elderly patients have a good support system at home, or that they have children who are willing to support them.

Now, let's move onto an even more complicated scenario.

Case Example 3

Mr. Tan was a 76-year-old man who came into the hospital after he developed fever for 3 days with lethargy. **He was found by his neighbours to be drowsy at the void deck.** *Blood profiles and chest X-ray revealed community-acquired pneumonia. His response to IV antibiotics was poor and antibiotics was escalated. His condition was complicated by poor compliance to fluid restriction as he also suffered from ERSF. His infection settled down on day 5 and the medical team intended to discharge him after completion of 7 days of IV antibiotics. However, the nursing team highlighted mobility and ADL difficulties as Mr. Tan required maximum assistance for transfers out of bed, and could not wear clothes without assistance. PT/OT was engaged to review patient but the patient could only tolerate sitting at the edge of bed. He remained unmotivated for rehabilitation due to his lower limb swelling and PT/OT was* **doubtful that he could return back to pre-morbid.** *His spouse who had been taking care of him and ensuring that he went to dialysis expressed* **caregiver stress** *as she was also getting older and needed her spouse to be independent because she was the only person taking care of him (she could not assist Mr. Tan's transfers to wheelchair by herself). She had* **financial concerns** *as well due to no insurance cover, a depleting MediSave reserve, and their children could barely support their own families, let alone to help them.*

Very often, when doctors and nurses encounter such issues, we will engage the MSW to assist in exploring possible solutions to transit patient back to the community. However, this compartmentalisation of responsibility often falls short in tackling the root of the problem. While the MSW can assist in looking for funds to help cover the hospitalisation fees, they would not know if compliance to fluid intake or diuretic medications help prevent another readmission. They would not be able to advise on appropriate mobility aids required to help Mr. Tan adapt and prevent falls (another admission to the hospital, albeit a different issue).

The examples illustrated above are just problems on the tip of the iceberg. There are many other issues like complex/chronic wounds, enteral feeding/tube access, palliative/end-of-life care issues, mobility problems, chronic diseases, home safety, and placement problems that are not explored here but may arise when you take care of these patients. Issues can be confounded and they may not present as *just one problem*.

To help you understand the myriad of non-medical issues out there, listed below are some of the commonly encountered problems.

Financial Issues	
	Locals Suggestions for possible solutions: • Subsidised rates for ward classes below 'A' • MediShield Life. This is a basic health insurance plan, administered by the Central Provident Fund (CPF) Board, which helps to pay for large hospital bills. All Singapore Citizens and Permanent Residents (PRs) are covered by MediShield Life. • Individual hospitalisation insurance plans. • Medical benefits from employment packages. • Subsidies and social funds may be available and subjected to approval should treatment or services be deemed necessary.
Inability to pay for hospitalisation fees and/or other services	

	• Patients who are unable to afford their medical bills after insurance coverage and MediSave utilisation can seek financial assistance from MSWs called MediFund. • Should patient require financial assistance for non-medical expenses, such as living expenses or employment, MSWs would be able to direct patients to Social Service Offices (SSO).
	Foreigners No subsidy. They have to pay the full amount of money during hospitalisation. Per day of hospitalisation can cost up to $300 SGD in 'C' class wards (without considering procedures or scans), hence treatments need to be considered wisely. • No MSW intervention applicable. Employees need to obtain letter of guarantee (LOG) from company to be processed by business office. Companies should have insurance cover for their employees up to a sum of money. • Foreign talents employed should have their individual staff medical benefits from employment packages. • Travellers or visitors may opt to continue treatment in their countries after their condition stabilises should they have no insurance cover.
Psychosocial issues	
Caregiver stress	Caring for their loved ones may be a noble desire but it may be unstainable or unsafe without proper support and training. Caregivers may express their concerns, fears, emotional burdens, and fatigue especially when there is an acute change in the functional abilities of their loved ones during hospitalisation.

	Suggestions for possible support:
	• Supportive counselling from MSW. • Caregiver training from various Allied Health. If the stress comes from an inability to cope with increased care needs, the next point can be further explored.
Inability to cope with increased care needs	Suggestions for possible solutions: • Rehabilitation programs (inpatient/outpatient) • Day care/Dementia day care • Foreign domestic helper • Home medical/nursing • Inpatient hospice • Nursing homes (government/private) *Solutions are not exhaustive, but listed to give a better idea.
Social/Placement Issues	Poor or no social support from family and/or community. Patient does not have any social support system to support their return to the community for a variety of reasons. There may be: • a lack of dedicated caregiver • strained relationships • home safety issues that may need help from social services. • abandonment of intellectually disabled/ vulnerable individuals during hospitalisation. • a lack of support and difficulty in securing placement to the available institutions/ residential home due to other unique circumstances. In the interim, restructured hospitals can be a temporary holding ground while their social and placement issues are sorted out.

Coping with Illness	Hospital admissions tend to be a life event when an individual is afflicted with a medical ailment. Difficulties with coping with life after illness may arise, be it care transition or emotional coping. Patients may require assistance with supportive counselling to help them progress past their medical event.

Table 2.5 Overview of Non-Medical Issues in Hospitals

While the above issues can add stress to the job demands of patient care, everyone in the healthcare team should help each other and **stop** passing the buck as it takes everyone in the healthcare team to help the patient. This is made even more important as the MOH's focus now is to move "beyond healthcare to home". To make this work in the community would require greater coordination and understanding of services available. As nurses, or any healthcare provider, you must care enough to help patients regain back their health and sense of confidence so that they can continue to live their lives meaningfully again back in their communities.

Referral to Allied Health

As you go for attachments and start working in the hospital, you will realise that a patient will also see many professionals from the allied health. Given the complexity of healthcare in today's world, health and wellness do not just fall on the shoulders of a single practitioner, but on a *team of capable healthcare providers*. It is important that as the facilitators of the patients' care, we know who to reach out to for their help and expertise.

However, with so many different personnel and activities seen on the wards, it may be difficult to fully appreciate the service and support that each profession of the allied health provides. Here is a list of services that is provided by the various allied health professionals.

REFER TO	COMMON SERVICES PROVIDED BY PROFESSION
Physiotherapist Care component: • **Gross mobility** • **Pain management** • **Respiratory care**	• Mobility assessment • Chest physiotherapy • Musculoskeletal pain management • Pre-operative physiotherapy • Gait retraining to assess fitness for discharge home • Gait aid training, if needed • Caregiver training • Post-operative rehabilitation • Stroke rehabilitation • Falls prevention *Outpatient setting* • Cardiac and pulmonary rehabilitation programmes • Chronic pain management • Sports rehabilitation • Osteoporosis clinics • Weight management • Vestibular rehabilitation
Occupational Therapist Care component: • **Activities of daily living**	• ADL/functional assessment • ADL retraining and modification • Identifying equipment needs and equipment prescription, if any (e.g. wheelchair, motorised scooter/ wheelchair) • Accessing the patient's home environment and provide home modification advice, if required • Falls prevention, energy conservation • Cognitive/activity engagement • Caregiver training • Splint and orthosis prescription

	Outpatient setting • Powered mobility aid training (e.g. motorised scooter) • Cognitive retraining • Hand and upper limb rehabilitation • Driving assessment and rehabilitation service (e.g. driving safety after recovering from physical deficits)
Speech Therapist Care component: • Swallowing • Communication	• Swallowing Disorders (e.g. dysphagia) • Voice Disorders (quality of voice inappropriate for an individuals' age, gender, cultural background) • Language Disorders (e.g. aphasia, dyslexia, dysgraphia) • Speech Disorders (apraxia of speech and dysarthria—most commonly as a result of stroke) • Fluency Disorders/Stuttering (interruption in flow of speaking)
Pharmacist Care component: • **Medication therapy management** • **Medication supplies**	• Medication reconciliation • Therapeutic dose monitoring (e.g. vancomycin dosing) • Verification of medication dosing • Therapy optimisation • Anticoagulation Clinic (ACC)–warfarin titration • Smoking cessation • Controlled drug supply • Procuring medication not in hospital formulary

Dietitian Care component: • **Nutrition support** • **Medical nutrition therapy** • **Chronic disease diet counselling**	• Assessment of nutrition status • Provides medical nutrition therapy for patients to correct or improve micronutrients derangements • Provides nutrition support via oral, enteral or parenteral route to meet nutritional requirements • Monitors compliance of inpatient therapeutic diets to established nutritional guidelines • Delivers nutrition education to empower patients to manage their chronic condition • Provides consultation to Food Service Department to ensure diets provided to inpatients are appropriate • Develops community and public health nutrition programs to promote health in the community
Podiatrist Care component: • **Foot ulcer management** • **Skin and nail care management** • **Musculoskeletal related**	• Active foot ulcer • Non-healing foot wounds • Foot wound infection • Prescribes footwears and accommodative insoles for offloading foot ulcers • Infected and painful ingrown toe nail *Outpatient setting* • Continued management from above inpatient referrals • Management of any existing PAD, neuropathy, and foot deformities (with or without wounds) • Diabetic foot care • Diabetic foot screening • General nail and skin care (painful corn and callus, verrucae, thickened nails, fungal infection) • Foot pain from musculoskeletal foot conditions (e.g. heel pain, bunion) • Gait analysis and orthotic therapy

Medical Social Worker	• Complex care and discharge planning, especially for patients who are physically and mentally disabled, frail elderly and children, with poor social support.
Care component: • **Care and discharge planning for poor, vulnerable populations** • **Psychosocial support** • **Financial support**	• Assisting in financial-related Issues (e.g. difficulties in affording medical bills and/ or living expenses) • Counselling and Therapy(e.g. coping with illness, grieve and bereavement, addiction issues) • Crisis Intervention and Risk-Assessment (e.g. domestic violence, suicide risk, drug overdose)

Table 2.6 Overview of Allied Health Services

Use this list of services wisely to guide you in caring holistically for your patients. As the main coordinator of patient's care, you hold the key to help physicians, patients and their families, and other professions know the most up-to-date and appropriate services for the individual.

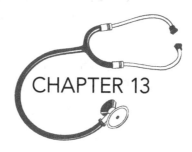

CHAPTER 13

NURSING DIAGNOSIS/CARE PLAN

In school, you are probably taught to use the North American Nursing Diagnosis Association (NANDA) list of nursing diagnosis to formulate your care plan for your patients. While that suggestion is great, there are so many diagnoses in the list that, as newbies, it would seem impossible to pick the right one for our patients.

To help you adapt faster, below is a list of what seems to be universal among all the different types of patients that come in everyday, regardless of any discipline that you are in.

GENERIC NURSING DIAGNOSES/CARE PLANS
- Acute/Chronic Pain
- Risk for Falls
- Risk of Infection
- Risk of Pressure Ulcer development
- Self-Care Deficit

To help you one step further, refer to the next few pages for a rapid assessment/algorithm to help you make a quick judgement of the nursing issues. Subsequently, you can add on more specific nursing issues from the basic set of care plans.

NURSING CARE PLAN QUICK ASSESSMENT

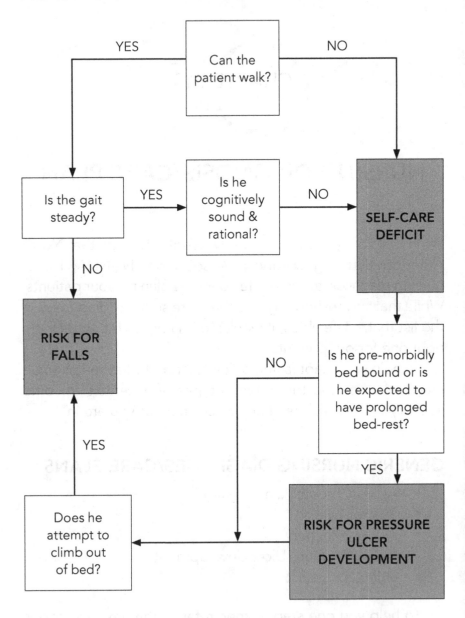

Table 2.7 Nursing Care Plan Quick Assessment (a)

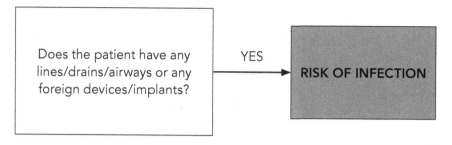

Table 2.8 Nursing Care Plan Quick Assessment (b)

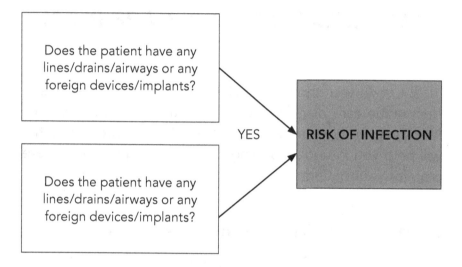

Table 2.9 Nursing Care Plan Quick Assessment (c)

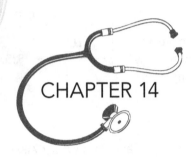

CHAPTER 14

FORMULATING YOUR CARE PLAN

By now, you should be all ready to take up cases and decide the care plan for each patient that you are in charge. Next, you will need to go through the thought processes that will help you in understanding and designing a specific care plan for your patients.

PRIMARY PROBLEM/CHIEF COMPLAINT

- What was/is the primary problem/chief complaint that brought the patient to the hospital?
- If he/she has been an inpatient for a while, what has already been done? What are the current treatment plans for him/her?
- Accompanying the primary problem, what would be the nursing issues that may arise?

When a patient comes into the hospital, it is expected that he/she will receive treatment. As the RN responsible for the patient, you need to know what is going on. If they had a complaint of moderate to severe pain somewhere, then it should be logical that there is at least a temporary solution (like having an IM Pethidine given STAT) for the pain if a permanent resolution cannot be met at that current juncture.

CO-MORBIDITIES AND PAST MEDICAL/ SURGICAL HISTORIES

- Other than the primary problem, what are the medical and surgical conditions (or anything else) that need to be taken note of?

Think in terms of the patient's chronic diseases (as discussed in 'Managing Chronic Diseases' subchapter under *Chapter 12: Taking Cases*). For example, patients with DM will need to have their blood sugars checked as they are prone to hyper- and hypoglycaemia. Also, for a patient with a stoma creation done many years ago after resection of colon cancer, nurses might still need to provide routine care of the stoma if the patient is unable to care for it by himself/herself.

NURSING ASSESSMENTS

- What would be the assessments that are crucial for the patient?

A head-to-toe assessment should be performed at every shift routinely. However, *highlight* assessments that are *important* and *relevant* to the primary problem. Document them in your progress notes. For instance, the lower limb neurovascular assessment of a patient with a right tibia fracture should demand closer attention and particular mention, as compared to that of a patient who has been admitted for pneumonia.

NURSING INTERVENTIONS AND MONITORING

- What are the nursing interventions that can be done, and what level of monitoring is required for each patient?

Following your nursing assessments, plan your interventions accordingly with the appropriate level of monitoring. If we have a patient that came back from surgery but is unable to participate much in physical activities, nurses can encourage and sit the patient out of bed at mealtimes as an intervention.

However, should his condition worsen and is now unable to sit out, nurses can then escalate their intervention and initiate 2-hourly turning and do regular perineum checks (especially if he is now bed bound with diapers) with other interventions as necessary.

DELIVERING TREATMENT

Link the treatment plans and what has been ordered by the physicians, as well as the inputs of the allied health professionals, to the patient's problem(s). All these plans should be aimed at progressing patients towards a goal of discharge.

While carrying out the treatment, think about the things that you are doing or not doing for the patient. Are they helping the patient? How to better help the patient?

- What is the frequency of the medications to be given to the patient? Are the frequency and dosage sufficient or too much? (e.g. is the volume of IV infusions ordered too much for a patient who is on fluid restriction?) Are there side effects that can be prevented? What are the possible adverse effects/side effects to be monitored for?

- Do the dressings need to be changed? How long later should the next change be? Are the wounds healing? If not, then why? And is there anything else that can be done?
- Are all the invasive lines working? Are they causing any problems? Do they need to be replaced? Have the lines fulfilled their purposes?
- Does the patient know what is going on? Do I need to educate him/her? Have all his/her concerns been addressed? Are the concerns realistic? Do I need to tweak his/her expectations?

FACILITATING TREATMENT PLANS

If you are not able to deliver the treatment, then you should facilitate for other professionals to come on board.

- Is the patient at his pre-morbid status? Is it appropriate to refer to the PT/OT now?
- Does the patient have a good nutritional status? Can the patient start to eat orally? Does he/she need a dietitian for nutritional support?
- Does the patient have difficulty in swallowing? Would a ST's recommendation be necessary?
- Is this radiological procedure available only during office hours? Can facilitate this procedure to be done earlier by getting ready earlier, or by calling the radiology/ intervention suite for an earlier slot?
- If treatments have been rendered, can I help to progress the patient to the next step of recovery?

Say if a patient underwent gastrectomy, nutrition replacement would be expected (either IV or per oral) and it would definitely be wise to monitor patient's intake and output strictly to make sure that he is not losing blood/fluids and taking in enough nutrition. If he/she does not eat well, and is not receiving IV nutrition, we then have to advocate for the patient. We can do this by alerting and discussing with the physicians and dietitians to re-formulate a plan so that he/she does not become malnourished in the process. It would then be our role to ensure that this information gets to the dietitian and physician so that a tailored made plan can be made for the patient.

DISCHARGE PLANNING: PATIENTS' TRANSITION BACK TO HOME/COMMUNITY
Section co-written with **Matthew Neo Ji Hui and Chew Tee Kit**

At any point in time of the hospitalisation from admission, think about how the patient will be going home. The end goal for the patient is always community re-integration. This can include patients at the end-of-life. Avoid resorting to institutionalisation of the patient as it should always be the last choice.

- Does the patient need a carer now? Was there a carer prior to admission? What is the carer's main purpose now?
- Are there new adaptations that the patient or carer needs to learn? Are they ready to start receiving caregiver training (CGT) now?
- Can the patient or carer cope with the new adaptation? Can they cope financially? Do they require MSW support?
- Is the CGT able to be completed during the patient's expected length of stay with more time or encouragement? Or would the patient require step-down care to allow a longer duration for CGT?

Note: Why this is important—many patients may **not** have had a carer at home. New carers, usually helpers or maids who have just arrived from overseas may be overwhelmed by the amount of responsibility they have which can affect any CGT that needs to be done.

- What are the services available out there in the community? Can they access these resources easily? Would they utilise the resources properly?
- Have all the appropriate team members come on board? Has any profession which would have been appropriate, been overlooked?

Discharge planning should occur from the time the patient is admitted, so that when the time comes, we would be able to discharge the patients back to the community with the appropriate training, skills, and resources in place. We *cannot expect* a patient with newly diagnosed DM to be able to perform a subcutaneous insulin injection in just one session. Once the patient is ready to learn, nurses should commence CGT even before the date of planned discharge is set.

Note that preparing a patient for discharge usually takes longer than expected as not all services in the hospital run 24/7. Services which run only during office hours such as most Allied Health services, or services which are more feasible to conduct during office hours such as CGT to the carer, or application for gait aids will have to be done early on. Buffer time to allow for patients and their family members or carers to learn the appropriate skills, or for paperwork for subsidies or application to other institutions of care to be processed. Hence, referring to the appropriate services **early** and notifying team members of expected timeframes to set everyone's expectations are hallmarks of good communication and will minimise confusion and frustration in the discharge planning process.

Furthermore, as discussed in the subchapter *"Managing Non-Medical Issues"*, health can be complicated by issues not related to medical issues. A good care plan needs to consider the patient's wishes, his/her and his/her family's resources, as well as the recommendations by various professions in the hospital.

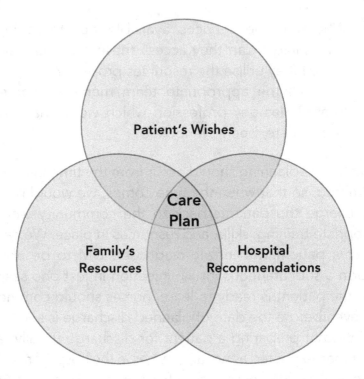

Table 2.10 Care Planning Venn Diagram

While considering and coordinating a care plan can be difficult, remember, your patients and their family members may sometimes express gratitude because they know that the plan is made in their best interests. The satisfaction from knowing that you have made a difference in their lives can be *priceless*.

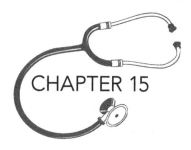

CHAPTER 15

WRITING GOOD DOCUMENTATION

Many students struggle with documentation and would spend a lot of time doing so. There are actually no hard rules when it comes to doing documentation. There are, however, some good principles that you should keep in mind when writing the patient's report.

Documentation, in general, should be:

- **Clear and concise.** They can be written in point forms. It is written to convey a message. Avoid "telling stories".
- **Chronologically written.** This will help the other healthcare professionals who are involved in the care of the patient to have a clear understanding of the flow of the events that happened.
- **Highlighting pertinent issues/assessments only.** If you embed important issues into an essay of various events that happened, chances of missing the important detail are a lot higher. If the patient has no issues other than the persistent pain over the abdomen, you could single out that particular issue, assess it, evaluate the treatments rendered and follow-up with a suggestion if it goes beyond your scope of care.

PROGRESS NOTES

This is the most commonly used note in your documentation. This is not just used by nursing, but also by medical and allied health, and whoever that has contact with patient. As the name suggests, anything that has to **PROGRESS** the patient's treatment and care forward can be classified here.

These could be your:

- **Nursing assessments** [including lines, tubes, drains, and wounds]. It could be during a dressing change when you realise that the wound is not healing, as the exudates are not well controlled. Write that down. If you feel that there's a need to switch product or escalate the management of the wound, highlight it.

- **Treatment rendered or omitted**. For instance, anti-hypertensives were omitted in view of low blood pressure of 105/60mmHg which deviates from baseline BP. Document. If it is persistent, you may want to get the doctor to follow-up on this.

- **Communication between medical team, allied health, the patients, and their family members**. A possible scenario could be that a physiotherapist recommended two weeks of inpatient rehabilitation in the morning. The patient's son came by in the morning and you conveyed physiotherapist's recommendation to him. The son then said that he would avail himself to help his father at home for two weeks instead of an inpatient rehabilitation service. As such, you documented the son's wish and suggest for a caregiver training (CGT) with the physiotherapist in the afternoon or the following day. The doctor took note of the communication and suggestion, and facilitated for the patient to go home after CGT is completed with patient's son.

Special mention: Document communication with Radiology department for scan timings—whether were are able to reach them, when is the scheduled timing/date, and what preparations are required so subsequent plans like surgical operation can follow suit. If the scan (or other preparations) is urgent, you may wish to also communicate verbally with relevant staff instead of only documenting in the notes.

- **Discharge planning.** Following the example above, you would understand that the patient could have deconditioned from prolonged hospital stay and would require the physiotherapist and occupational therapist's clearance during this admission when he is well enough to engage in such activity. As a nurse, you can make an input such as: "*Suggest to refer to PT/OT as the patient is currently not safe for home*".

In general, it is good to follow in the format of **SOAP** (**S**ubjective, **O**bjective, **A**ssessment, **P**lan) in writing your shift summary in your progress note. Even if the headings that your organisation adopts are different, the flow of writing and the thought process can follow this format.

CARE PLAN

Typically formatted and written as **APIE** (**A**ssessment, **P**roblem, **I**ntervention, **E**valuation). If the risk of infection is a problem for the patient due to the presence of IV cannula, then the intervention can be to assess for phlebitis. The evaluation can be: "*Redness seen over right antecubital fossa cannula site with some pain upon administering IV medication. Risks of possible phlebitis explained to patient and IV cannula removed. To continue monitoring for resolution of phlebitis.*"

FLOW SHEETS/CHARTS

Flow sheets are simple to use and update. Our role is to make sure that they are updated accurately per shift so that when there is an issue, we can trace back when the changes started to occur. Some of these sheets are also checklists.

Checklists can help us to remember important steps and things to consider when doing a procedure, especially if you are unfamiliar when the procedure. Commonly used checklists include nursing assessment, lines/tubes/drains, intake/output, and daily cares/safety. Also, pull out and fill up charts relevant to individual patients, for example, a pre-op checklist for the patient that is going for surgery, or a blood administration checklist for the patient requiring blood a transfusion.

Example of a Typical Acute Care Patient with a Well-Documented Care Plan

Background

A 55-year-old male was admitted for poorly healing ulcer of the right big toe. Significant past medical history includes DM hypertension and hyperlipidaemia. Ultrasound Doppler was done during the previous shift and the medical team decided to plan for right lower limb angiogram and angioplasty in the afternoon.

Medical Inputs
Vascular AM Rounds S/B Senior Consultant @ 0830H Patient alert, sitting out of bed Heart – S1S2 Lungs – Clear Abdomen – Soft, non-tender Calves – supple Right lower limb – right big toe dorsum 2x2cm ulcer, sloughy. Dressing stained with yellow discharge.

Issues:

1. Non-healing right big toe ulcer b/g DM, HTN, HLD

- US findings:
Right LL: > 75% stenosis of the superficial femoral artery

Discussed with the patient and offered angioplasty. Indication: to improve blood supply to the leg, improve chances of healing for right big toe ulcer. Risks of surgery including contrast-induced nephropathy (CIN) explained. Patient consented. Site marked.

Plan:

- NBM now
- Listed for R LL angiogram, angioplasty in EOT under MAC today
- Q4H SCSI, Q4H BGM
- Renal Panel STAT
- Hold off enalapril (risk of Acute Kidney Injury)
- IV N-Acetylcysteine (NAC) now (to prevent CIN)
- Start IV NaCl 0.9% 2L/24h

After reading this, you carry out all the changes. You also received a call from the OT saying that the operation is scheduled at 4 p.m.

Nursing Inputs

Care Plan:

Risk of infection: monitor for phlebitis—redness and swelling.
Evaluation: Nil signs of infection seen over IV plug.
Monitor for right big toe wound deterioration – Nil
surrounding redness and swelling. Peri-wound not warm to
touch.
Evaluation: No suspicion of spreading infection.

Risk for falls: advised patient to call for help if he needs to
move about.
Evaluation: call bell within reach, patient able to call for help
as needed.

Shift Summary

S -
Patient alert, generally well. Slightly anxious for operation,
assured patient.
IV plug inserted over the left arm, Renal Panel taken and IV
hydration started.
Nil c/o pain over right big toe wound. Dressings intact, not
soaked.
Rationale for NBM emphasised to patient. Advised patient
to safe keep his belongings prior to OT.

O -
T: 36.3
BP: 110/66
HR: 81
RR: 17
SPO2: 99%

A -
Right big toe wound stable

P -

- NBM since 0900h, await Op at 1600h. Site marked by the team.
- Enalapril morning dose withheld
- Continue IV hydration
- Continue neurovascular assessment

Example of a Deteriorating Patient with a Well-Documented Care Plan

Background (Follow-up from the previous case)

A 55-year-old male was admitted for ulcer of the right big toe from the emergency department. Significant past medical history includes DM, hypertension, and hyperlipidaemia. Pre-operatively, the patient received IV hydration 2L/24h. The patient underwent R LL angiogram angioplasty in EOT under MAC (monitored anaesthesia care) and came back to the ward. He appeared breathless after an hour of coming back to the ward and now requires increased supplemental O2 to maintain Spo2 > 95%.

He was reviewed by the on-call House Officer who ordered for ECG, cardiac enzymes and portable CXR. The CXR shows haziness in bilateral bases and the on-call House Officer mentions that he is concerned about fluid overload.

Nursing Inputs

Noted patient's SPO2 desat to 90% on 2L nasal prongs, accompanied with SOB

Was on O2 via 2L nasal prongs since back from OT.

GCS 15 – E4V5M6
Vitals -
T: 38.0
BP: 110/59
HR: 100
RR: 29
SPO2: 90% on 2L nasal prongs, increased to 98% on 5L simple face mask

New onset of SOB and desaturation needing increased O2 supplementation.
Informed Dr. Goh STAT to review patient. Escalated to 5L simple face mask.

Shift Summary

S -
Noted patient breathless and desaturated while on 2L nasal prongs. O2 delivery was escalated to 5L via simple face mask with Spo2 improving to 98%. Dr. Goh was informed. CXR and ECG performed. IDC was inserted by Dr. Goh for strict I/O monitoring. STAT bloods were taken. IV hydration was discontinued, and IV Furosemide was given.

O -
Vitals as above

A -
Possible fluid overload

P - Hourly vitals, urine output monitoring Keep Spo2 > 95% as per team STOP IV Hydration (MAR hold for now, team kindly discontinue if not needed) Keep patient's wife updated
Communication Note Was approached by patient's wife at the nursing counter. She was concerned as she noticed her husband was now on face mask and had IDC inserted. • Informed her that the doctors felt that her husband could have developed fluid accumulation in his lungs. • Currently he is being closely monitored and we are watching his response to the medication that was given to help remove the fluids from his lungs. The IDC allows closer monitoring of his fluid status. • Our doctors will update her when they can. • Patient's wife appreciated the updates and would like to be kept updated on the progress. • Team kindly update when able to.

LEARNING POINTERS

Good documentations are in short, **FOCC.**

- **Focused.** It serves a purpose of progressing the patient towards discharge. It also surfaces potential problems and hindrances. It highlights issues revolving around the *patient*, and is not the place to vent about internal hospital issues or processes.
- **Objective.** Does not exaggerate or underplay the issues. It is also formal in writing and hence the usage of personal pronoun tends to be omitted. Personal

pronoun is used in situations where advocacy is adopted.

- **Concise.** It summarises the encounters into important points essential for the healthcare team members to take note. It does not contain unnecessary verbal communication or irrelevant assessments and repeated points.
- **Clear.** It does not confound multiple issues into a single piece. It should be readable and the main points can be captured instantly. Should an action or follow-up be required from someone in the healthcare team, it can be highlighted in bold to guide the reader to capture the main point(s) faster in a sea of information and words.

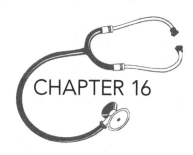

CHAPTER 16

REVIEW AND SELF-ASSESSMENT

1. A 60-year-old male came in for suspected intestinal obstruction. Upon arrival, he started vomiting green, bilious fluids. An NGT was then inserted and you aspirated out green fluids until no more fluid can be aspirated. The patient felt instant relief. He is alert and orientated to his surroundings. The immediate nursing care that follows should include:

   A. Chest X-Ray to confirm placement of NGT
   B. NBM and nurse head up at least 30 degrees to prevent pulmonary aspiration.
   C. Monitor nasal mucosal lining 4 hourly for signs of mucosal erosion.
   D. Put patient on hand mittens to prevent accidental removal of NGT.

2. You receive a call from the HDU that a patient with a tracheostomy tube size 6 (un-cuffed, non-fenestrated) is coming to your cubicle as he is stable enough to be nursed in the general ward. The most important action to do would be to:

A. Put him on continuous vitals monitoring as soon as he reaches the ward.
B. Inform your preceptor and your nurse doing the junior role of the incoming admission.
C. Standby a trachy dilator, humidifier unit, oxygen tank, suction apparatus and vital monitoring ready by the bedside.
D. Prepare a tracheostomy kit (trachy dilator, pressure manometer), a same-sized and a smaller-sized cuffed non-fenestrated tube and suction apparatus ready by the bedside.

3. *A routine check of your patient's NGT revealed that it has been more than two weeks since its insertion. The patient had a Ryle's tube inserted after being admitted for an acute stroke and is still undergoing rehabilitation in the general ward. You would then:*

A. Discuss with the physicians whether it is appropriate to change the NGT as it has expired.
B. Suggest changing to a flexiflo/corflo (silicone NGT) as it is softer and can last longer.
C. Pull out the NGT immediately and raise a report.
D. Continue to monitor for mucosal breakdown. Look at Speech Therapist's and Dietitian's recommendations or discuss with them. Continue using the existing tube if the patient is progressing well with swallowing and does not have any signs of mucosal breakage in his nose.

4. *A patient who had been kept NBM for OGD has now been allowed to eat after the scopes. The scope findings were normal, and the patient appeared well and comfortable during his post-procedure review by the House Officer. He has a background of DM, ESRF*

and previous cholecystectomy. He weighs about 60kg with a height of 165cm. He should be allowed:

A. Diet of choice, low fat, low salt, low potassium, low phosphate and 2000kCal DM diet.
B. Minced diet, low fat, low salt, low potassium, and 1500kCal DM diet.
C. Diet of choice, low fat, low salt, low potassium, and 1500kCal DM diet.
D. Diet of choice, low potassium, low phosphate, and 2000kCal DM diet.

5. *You are informed by your junior nurse that the patient's BSL is 3.7mmol/L. The patient is alert, conversant, and asymptomatic. You will:*

A. Inform physician STAT. Suggest for physician to order PO Dextrose 15g to correct the hypoglycaemia. In the meantime, serve the patient with a cup of milo.
B. Standby IV dextrose-saline. Inform physician and wait for the order before administering.
C. Serve PO dextrose 15g in 100ml of water. Recheck hypo-count in 15mins and inform the physician. Monitor patient closely and document outcome.
D. Serve any sweetened drinks available on patient's cardiac table. Then prepare IV Dextrose 50% for the doctor to administer in case the patient becomes unconscious.

Questions 6 & 7 share the same patient history.

6. *You receive a patient from the Emergency Department (ED) and he was transferred from a trolley to bed. Continuous IV Nexium is running on his right arm. He greets you with a smile and asks for a urinal as he is*

feeling too weak to ambulate to the toilet. He appears skinny. The ED Nurse tells you that he came in for upper gastro-intestinal bleed with melaena stools x 3 days. Your immediate nursing care plan should identify him as:

A. Self-care deficit, risk for falls, and risk for infection.
B. Risk for falls, risk for pressure ulcer development, and risk for infection.
C. Self-care deficit, risk for pressure ulcer development, and risk for infection.
D. Risk for falls, risk for infection, and acute/chronic pain.

7. *The previous patient you received from the ED has now come back from emergency oesophago-gastro-duodenoscopy (OGD) and still has ongoing melaena. He has been given three units of blood since admission. During diaper changing, he complains of prickly pain around the perianal area. You also noticed some redness around the scrotum. You should:*

A. Raise incident report and inform ward sister. Subsequently do regular potting and document observation.
B. Suspect incontinence-associated dermatitis and inform doctor. Suggest use of an anal plug.
C. Start application of barrier cream and a temporary urinary sheath. Document observation and monitor perineum at least once per shift. Highlight to the next shift to do more regular diaper checks.
D. Start cradle nursing and apply foam dressing to sacrum.

8. *Inspection of an IV cannula on a patient revealed redness along the cannula and pain on touch. The IV cannula is a day old. IV Augmentin and IV Paracetamol need to be administered later.*

A. Since phlebitis score is +2, we should advise the patient that re-siting of the cannula is required, as it is likely to develop to +3 with continued use.

B. Although phlebitis score is +2, we can just continue monitoring. Remove the IV cannula only if the patient cannot tolerate.

C. Since phlebitis score is +1, it is okay to use the cannula with careful monitoring and advise the patient that the redness and pain are temporary.

D. Although phlebitis score is +1, we are able to proceed with infusion if the patient can tolerate.

9. *A 79-year-old male has a past medical history of DM, HTN, HLD and ESRF. Today is his POD 4 for total colectomy. Physiotherapists have only managed to sit him at the edge of bed once yesterday. After physical therapy today, your junior nurse informs you that his heart rate is 119BPM. You should:*

A. Check if the patient has any other complaints. Proceed to check a full set of vitals. If patient is asymptomatic, and the heart rate comes down to baseline, it may be exertion related tachycardia. Inform the physician of the full set of vitals and your assessment.

B. Suspect fluid overload causing pulmonary oedema and suggest that the physician take a set of ABG for diagnosis.

C. Suspect pulmonary embolism due to prolonged bed rest. Inform physician STAT.

D. Suspect progression shock secondary to hypovolaemia. The patient may be dehydrated from high output stoma, post-op bleeding, and recent exercise. Suggest commencing IV fluid replacement immediately.

10. A patient presses the call bell and complains that he is feeling giddy on the bed. He looks slightly lethargic. He is fearful that something might be wrong so he asks you to inform the doctor. You checked the vitals two hours ago and it revealed BP: 105/60mmhg, HR: 95bpm, O2 saturation: 100%, T: 37.0 °C. You also checked the BSL, which was 5.5mmol/L one hour ago. You will:

A. Assure the patient that he is okay, as his latest set of vitals were still within the normal range. The nursing team will check on him again later during the next routine vitals check and escalate if necessary.

B. Inform physician that the patient complained of giddiness and convey the vitals taken two hours ago. Suggest reviewing the patient.

C. Recheck vital signs now and assess the patient at the same time. Check fluid balance. Compare with baseline and inform physicians about any complications you may suspect.

D. Set IV plug immediately and standby for possible deterioration. Inform your junior nurses to keep a close eye on the patient for the rest of the shift.

Answers

1. **B.** The purpose of inserting the NGT is to decompress the gastric contents to allow bowel rest. Allowing diet in this case would defeat this purpose and likely induce vomiting. Elderly patients are at even higher risk of aspirating from vomitus due to the poorer gag-reflex. They are also prone to developing aspiration pneumonia. B is the most appropriate answer. While CXR is necessary to confirm placement of NGT, being able to aspirate a large amount of bilious fluids can be indicative of right placement. A simple pH test would suffice. Mucosal erosion is a possible complication, but since the NGT is newly inserted, the urgency is not with such a monitoring. Hand mittens are only considered if the patient is non-compliant with his safety.

2. **D.** The most important thing in receiving a patient with tracheostomy is to prepare the necessary equipment in case of dislodgment. Simply informing colleagues (doctors, nurses) of the incoming admission does not translate into actual nursing care. Answer C is a close option but does not adequately prepares for a reinsertion. A cuffed and smaller sized tracheostomy tube is necessary as newly formed tracheostomies usually have plenty of secretions and the stoma tract has not been well-established. Cuffed tubes help patient to breathe fully through the tube.

3. **D.** There is currently no literature which supports routine change in NGT as there are no specific expiry dates. There is, however, literature that suggests that every NGT insertion poses new risks of developing complications like aspiration pneumonia, trauma, etc. Since this patient is still undergoing rehabilitation and has a chance of being weaned off NGT, it is wise to reduce cost and trauma to patient by keeping the NGT

in situ while monitoring for mucosal breakage. There is no immediate need to switch to a softer, "longer term" NGT. Therefore, D is the most appropriate answer as it considers the patient as a whole and not just the "problem".

4. **A.** There is no mention of swallowing deficits, hence there is no reason why the patient needs to have a minced diet and cannot have DOC. Answer B is out. Patients with previous cholecystectomy should avoid high-fat diet as this may induce loose stools. Answer D is out. The remaining answers A & C are very similar, but answer A is the better answer. Consider the BMI of the patient (BMI 22), which is within the healthy range. Having 2000kcal maintains his energy requirements. ESRF patients should generally be on low salt diet (to prevent fluid retention), as well as low potassium and low phosphate diet (as they have impaired renal excretion of potassium and phosphate).

5. **C.** While informing the physician is important, rectifying the problem before it progresses is more important. As the hypo-count in the question is not dangerously low, and the patient is not drowsy, as RNs we should be able to resolve such issues quite competently as IV dextrose is not needed yet at this stage. Nurses are allowed to order and give oral dextrose as per protocol. We should also never attempt to resolve hypoglycaemia with milo alone, as it is a complex sugar that takes longer time to be converted and absorbed in the gut. The most appropriate answer is therefore C.

6. **A.** The patient seems rational and cognitively sound— he knows that he should not walk now because he is feeling weak. He is at risk for falls as his gait is unlikely to be steady due to the loss of blood. Because he cannot walk much now, he has some self-care deficit, especially in elimination. He is however not at risk of developing

pressure ulcers at this current juncture because he is able to ask for help and likely able to turn himself. With an IV plug, he is at risk of developing infection. A is the best answer. In reality, however, you will not be faulted for including risk of developing pressure ulcer in your care plan.

7. **C.** The prickly pain is a sign of worsening incontinence-associated dermatitis. The best way to restore skin condition is through moisture reduction (urinary sheath to divert urine) and skin-barrier application to protect the skin against faeces. Regular potting will not be effective, as skin will continue to break down. Use of anal plug is not effective against large amounts of loose stools as leakage may still happen. Use of foam dressing alone may also not be effective as high chance of seepage to the dressing can be expected. C is the best answer.

8. **A.** Presence of pain and streak formation correspond to a +2 on the visual infusion phlebitis score. Answers C and D are out. If a +2 score is present, it is essential to advise patient to re-site the cannula, as the chance of worsening phlebitis is high. Answer B is out as we should not leave a culprit IV cannula in situ when we have already suspected phlebitis.

9. **A.** While answers B to D are possible reasons why patients can have tachycardia, jumping to these conclusions may not be helpful. A full set of vitals is more useful than just a single parameter. A good RN also needs to be able to interpret vital signs competently. Simply informing the physicians about abnormal vital signs without any thought process does not reflect well on our profession. Of course, if you do have concerns about the patient's safety, do not hesitate to highlight your concerns to the physicians. And do not forget, be cautious with fluid therapy in patients with ESRF!

10. **C.** Answer B is out as the nurse merely acts as a middleman between the patient and the doctor. Answer A may be a good answer, but the nurse did not take any updated parameters before coming to that conclusion. Answer D, is acting blindly without addressing the patient's complaints or further investigating the situation. It is possible that this patient may be slowly progressing towards hypovolaemic shock as his latest set of vitals show borderline tachycardia and borderline low blood pressure. Taking a new set of vitals and fluid balance may provide a clearer picture of what is going on. If the giddiness persists, even if the vital signs are in the normal range, do inform the physician for review, as it is not normal to experience prolonged giddiness while resting.

AFTERWORD

Remember, you are *not* just doing what your preceptor tells you to do. You are also *not* just clearing your competency checklists. You are a nurse-in-training. You should be putting on your thinking cap when you are out in the placement areas. Think about how to care for the patient from admission to discharge to the community. Aim for minimal guidance from your preceptor. If possible, aim for **collaboration**.

The journey in nursing can be very daunting, but with the right tools I believe that you will make it through just fine. I also believe that you have chosen this profession because there is something inside you that wants to do more.

Remember, *"the eye sees only what the mind knows"*. As you know and understand more, you will slowly realise that you will be able to see things that you could not see before. Keep learning and be humble to acquire knowledge even in the unlikeliest of people or places.

Now, go forth and strive to be the best that you can be!

Printed in the United States
By Bookmasters